Chic & Slim
TOUJOURS

AGING
BEAUTIFULLY
LIKE THOSE
CHIC
FRENCH
WOMEN

Anne Barone

THE ANNE BARONE COMPANY

Chic & Slim Toujours: Aging Beautifully Like Those Chic French Women
Anne Barone

A Chic & Slim Book
Published by The Anne Barone Company, Texas 76309 USA

ISBN: 978-1-937066-09-3
Printed in the United States of America

Book and Cover Design: Anne Barone
Chic Woman Image Copyright © iStockphoto/ Yordanka Poleganova
Eiffel Tower Design: Joyce Wells GriggsArt

This book is intended as philosophy and general reference only. It is not to be used as a substitute for medical advice or treatment. Every individual's problems with the aging process are unique and complex. You should consult your physician for guidance on any medical condition or health-issues and to make sure any product or treatment you use are right and safe for you. The author and publisher disclaim any responsibility for any liability, loss or risk incurred directly or indirectly from the use or application of any of the contents of this publication or from any of the materials, machines, services or products mentioned in it.

Mention of specific companies, products, organizations or authorities in this book does not imply endorsement by the author or publisher, nor does mention of specific companies, products, organizations or authorities imply that they endorse this book, its author, or its publisher. Every effort has been made that internet addresses and other sources of information are accurate at the time of publication.

For more links and related information visit:
http://www.annebarone.com

Contents

The further into your 60s you are,
the harder it is to look 29.
Not impossible. Just more difficult.

Maintaining a healthy, attractive appearance from the time your body begins its mid-life changes into advanced senior years takes more effort than in those youthful days when, with a pair of jeans that fit well, a suntan and a skin care routine that involved soap and water, you looked just great. Over 50, jeans may not suit your personal style. The sun will likely cause age spots. An attractive older face may require a tad more attention than just quick cleansing.

Despite the challenges, French women age remarkably well. They continue to be chic and slim, successful in their careers and romantically active into their 70s and beyond. My *Chic & Slim* system is a works-wherever-you-live translation of techniques I learned from chic French women.

In this *Chic & Slim* book we look at techniques chic French women employ to become those magnificent *femmes d'un certain âge. Toujours.* Forever.

be chic, stay slim *toujours* — Anne Barone

Femmes d'un Certain Âge

The French, known for *politesse* and diplomacy, do not say an older woman, nor a middle-aged woman, nor specify a woman's decade, they say a woman is *"un femme d'un certain âge."* A woman of a certain age.

We now use the translated phrase in English. In novels written in English in the 1920s and 1930s, you can also find the phrase "a woman of uncertain age." The woman of certain—or uncertain—age is one who is no longer young, but without knowing her real age, you would have difficulty guessing it. She has taken such excellent care of herself and has such wonderful charm and chic, she may be older than she looks, but her real age does not matter. That is the sort of certain age that concerns us in this book.

The majority of the chic women of certain age I discuss in this book are over 50. The youngest is 43. Oldest is 99, healthy, active and chic. Ages 43 to 99 give us a span of 56 years. At age 66 as I complete this book, I view certain age from the perspective of much experience with this life stage.

With *Chic & Slim Toujours* you can age beautifully just like those chic French *femmes d'un certain âge.*

About the Author Anne Barone

Once fat and frumpy, in her mid-20s Anne Barone began to learn chic French women's techniques for eating well and staying slim and for dressing chic on a small budget. She lost 55 pounds and acquired a chic French wardrobe.

Chicer and slimmer, Anne Barone returned to the USA to find a nation growing sloppier and fatter. She decided to share her French secrets. In 1997, Anne Barone published her first French-inspired book *Chic & Slim: how those chic French women eat all that rich food and still stay slim.* More *Chic & Slim* books followed. The latest book *Chic & Slim Toujours: aging beautifully like those chic French women* reveals French secrets for dressing chic and staying slim in a woman's middle and later years.

Now 66, Anne Barone lives in Texas where she is attempting to create a bit of French Provence on the North Texas plains. "Far enough in the country to grow eggplant, apricots and lavender. But close enough to Dallas to make the sales at Neiman Marcus."

You can learn more about Anne Barone and *Chic & Slim* at the companion website *annebarone.com*

MORE CHIC & SLIM BOOKS
by Anne Barone

Chic & Slim: how those chic french women eat
all that rich food and still stay slim

Chic & Slim Encore: more about how
french women dress chic stay slim—and
how you can too!

Chic & Slim Techniques: 10 techniques
to make you
chic & slim *à la francaise*

Using Toujours for Success

Chic & Slim Toujours begins with those well-cut chic French hairstyles and works down to the toes of those sexy stiletto-heeled shoes. The book then looks at chic French women's approach to food, exercise and stress that keeps them slim at ages when chic women in many other countries see their bathroom scale numbers climb. We consider chic French women of certain age at work, as well as how they maintain their mystique, their relationships and their incomparable personal styles.

Since most of you reading this book live elsewhere than France, the information is designed to give you chic French results no matter where you live. You will find additional useful information on the *Chic & Slim* website *annebarone.com*.

Many of the chic French women in the book are those you have admired for years. Unless you live in or spend much time in France, however, the names of others may not be familiar. But you will enjoy meeting these interesting women and getting to know more about them. The women in these page represent a variety of ages, careers, ethnic backgrounds, and varieties of French chic.

Approach *Chic & Slim Toujours* as you would the menu in a French bistro. Not everything on the menu may be to your taste, this is, your personal style and lifestyle. But no matter your age, career, income level, ethnic background, or personal style, you will surely find something delicious.

Bon appétit!

With freedom and honor

you should be your own sculptor

to fashion your form as you choose

Pico della Mirandola

Hair

THE MORNING OF MY 33RD BIRTHDAY I looked in the mirror and saw three gray hairs. I plucked them out. That took care of that. At least for a few more years. But I could not prevent the inevitable: with certain age arrives more changes in our hair than just a little gray. Those changes require changes in response: in hair care products, often in our hair's style and length. They require decisions about hair color. Yes or no? If yes, natural or new?

And if, as chic French women believe, our personal style sends a message as to who we are and what we are about, then, as our lives move into this new stage, we may want to send an updated message.

In *Mirror, Mirror: The Terror of Not Being Young*, Elissa Melamed quotes an anonymous certain age woman who says, "I am prepared to die, but not to look lousy for the next forty years." Chic French women did not look lousy the first 40 years and they don't intend to look lousy the last 40 years, nor any years between. When aging presents challenges to maintaining beautiful hair, chic French women take action. Often this action includes expert professional help and advice.

Christophe Robin, the Parisian colorist who cares for the tresses of such chic French women of certain age as Catherine Deneuve,

Isabelle Adjani, and Fanny Ardant, has this to say about women's hairstyle and color:

> Young women in their 20's can be excessive and original because of the freshness of their complexion and eyes. At 30, a women should resolutely define her style. The 40 year old woman should do everything possible to soften and add sex appeal to her look. At 50, a woman should do her maximum to seem younger, to have shiny, well cared for hair. She should also be careful about keeping her complexion and style from becoming dull or boring.

Good news today that we have such a huge arsenal of products and techniques and talented *artistes des cheveux*, not only in France, but in almost every country of the world, that with a little effort and money, we can have that shiny, healthy, well-cared-for hair perfect for our personal style. Useful, perhaps, for us to look at a number of chic French women who are no longer young, but still very attractive, and see what ideas we might gather from their hairstyle and hair color choices.

Note: You may find it useful to see photos of the women I am discussing. You can find them online. Many of these chic French women have a website or Wikipedia page. Some have Wikipedia pages in both French and English. Google Images will bring up photos of most of these women, though recent photos might be scattered among others from decades ago.

A quick survey of chic French certain age hairstyles today might suggest that the principal choice is between natural gray cut short, or shoulder length in that popular reddish-brown shade that I think of as French Certain Age Mahogany. A more detailed examination, however, shows chic French women choose a range of lengths, styles and hair colors. True, blond is not as frequent a choice as the darker shades. But one of the best known chic French women Catherine Deneuve, 67, early in her film career made a personal style decision for long and blond, as it remains today. Yet in 1992 *Elle* magazine featured an interview with French fashion designer Yves Saint-Laurent "30 Years of YSL." The accompanying Andre Rau photographs of fashions from YSL's various collections were modeled by Catherine Deneuve. Her hair in these photos is a short dark cap dramatically highlighted. I was surprised by the change from her usual long blond hairstyle. Once chic French women define their personal style, they do not usually make radical alteration in both color and length. Catherine Deneuve looked beautiful. But not quite Catherine Deneuve. In any case, the next time I saw Catherine Deneuve in a media photograph, her hair was again that luxurious to-the-shoulders blond hair. A lesson here that you can experiment with new hair colors and hair cuts with the freedom to return to your previous style or move on to another if you don't like the results.

Another chic French woman of certain age who chooses blond, though a darker, more subtle shade than Catherine Deneuve, is Anne Lauvergeon, 51, the CEO of AREVA, a French energy conglomerate chiefly concerned with nuclear power. In recent years her hairstyle choice was long, flipping out softly around the shoulders of her chic suits. She wore a side part and thick bangs. Subtle highlights gave her a dark blonde shade. A recent photo in *Forbes* magazine's 100 Most Powerful Women in the World series, shows that her long hair has been trimmed to a sleeker, just-above-the-shoulders length, though the bangs, side part and highlights remain. Photographers are often attracted, not to Anne Lauvergeon's hair, but to her great legs on display between her stiletto heels and the hems of those pencil skirts of her chic suits she wears.

Chic French women whose natural hair color is black very often stick with that color in certain age. Jewelry designer, Paloma

Picasso, 61, currently celebrating 30 years association with Tiffany is a beautiful example continuing the mid-length jet black shade that was so captivating in those striking and sophisticated red and black magazine ads for her Paloma Picasso fragrance.

Another chic French woman of certain age who has retained her black hair color in certain age is Anne Cheng, 55, Chair of Intellectual History of China at the College de France and authority on Confucianism. Born in Paris to Chinese parents, Anne Cheng's classic Oriental beauty is shown to advantage by the reds and blacks she often wears. Anne Cheng wears her cap of dark hair with a center part full at top and sides. An attractive style for a busy academic teaching and lecturing on a schedule that involves international travel.

Tatiana de Rosnay, 48, has glorious shoulder length naturally gray hair. This author of *Elle s'appelait Sarah*, (English title: Sarah's Key) told the interviewer for *Madame Figaro* that she began to gray at 19 and from 20 to 40 she colored her hair. Then she stopped and made her gray hair her trademark. She pampers those gray hairs with *Shampooing Éclat Silver de L'Oréal Professionnel* and John Frieda Frizz Ease. Plus, she says, she spends a *lot* of time at her hairdresser's because she wants her hair always to look perfect.

Another whose chic is augmented by gray hair is Michèle Alliot-Marie, 64. President Nicholas Sarkozy's first Minister of Defense, also served as Justice and Foreign Ministers. The French call her *"la dame en fer,"* Iron Lady, for her often brusque, no-nonsense manner. Her current hairstyle lays a soft wave across her forehead and gives her a more feminine appearance than the short cap she wore in earlier certain age. The updated, softer hairstyle works well with her rimless eyeglasses. The more feminine hairstyle also coordinates better with her body type. She is more generously endowed in the bust than many French woman, and she has great legs she shows off in pencil shirts and high heels. Michèle Alliot-

Marie is an extremely chic dresser. On election night when the women of the new French government lined up across the stage with the new French president, her outfit captured the most chic prize in that tough chic French women competition.

Christine Albanel, 55, who served as France's Culture Minister from 2007 until 2009, is in the medium-to-dark brown hair with subtle highlights camp. Looking over media photos of the past several years, you find slight variations in depth of color and length. All looked attractive. Christine Albanel's haircut is basically the one I currently wear: a chin length bob with side part and bangs. When cut well and trimmed regularly, it is an easy maintenance style. Just wash with a good quality shampoo and pamper it with a conditioning treatment and let it air dry. French women generally prefer not to use heat appliances on their hair, nor spend the time that blowing dry requires. My preference is the same. Though when the haircut begins to grow out and you don't have time for a trim that week, or when you want a more formal look, a little attention with a curling iron or hot rollers will improve your look.

France is almost synonymous with Culture. As Culture Minister, Christine Albanel had a demanding schedule with appearances at many important formal affairs, as she had in her previous job as president of the Museum and Domaine of Versailles. Her hairstyle looked as appropriate when she was dressed in formal French designs as in chic workday pant suits or in casual clothes.

Times past it was a style truism in the USA that women of a certain age should not wear long hair—at least not unless it was secured in a neat bun or elegant chignon. Chignon by the way, derives from the French phrase *chignon du cou*, nape of the neck. Long hair was thought to "pull the face down," when Nature was already pulling the face down more than a woman wanted. Puritanical attitudes in the USA frowned on long hair as a little too sexy and youthful for certain age women. Shouldn't they be over that? French women don't think one is ever too old to look sexy. Too, today with all the "medical editing" of signs of aging available and wonderful hair products and easy access to information of hair care and style ideas, women in their 40s and older can look marvelous with long hair. For women in certain age, looking attractive in long hair simply depends on color, style, health of hair, the wearer's skin tone. And I would add, the personality of the woman wearing the long hair.

While chic French women often choose longer hairstyles as far into certain age as their 80s, both the bun and chignon can be elegant and time-saving options. Today a wonderful example of the bun is the one of rich mahogany brown hair worn by Simone Veil, 83, a French lawyer and Nazi concentration camp survivor, who when French Health Minister in the 1970s, pushed for major improvements in women's health that make French women's lives easier today. The French have long admired Simone Veil's beauty and courage. Her hairstyle choice is a regal one befitting a grande dame of French politics and culture who now occupies a seat of the *Académie française*, only the sixth woman to serve this prestigious body since its creation in 1635.

In decades of her films we have seen the dark black hair of French actress Isabelle Adjani, 55. Lately her hair has taken on a rich mahogany hue. Reportedly she is a client of hair color guru Christophe-Robin. At the latest Cannes awards we saw Isabelle Adjani with long flowing locks. Was the length helped with hair extensions? Like the shorter chignon style, hair pieces are extremely useful for giving a woman both everyday convenience of shorter hair and long for more elegant evenings.

In Isabelle Adjani's case, the question of extensions arises because in her most recent film, she is seen with a short, unglamorous style that definitely suits her character. She plays a teacher in a tough school where on a bad day she shoots one of her students and takes her class hostage at gunpoint. Oh dear! In my childhood, my idea of a French school teacher was that nice nun that shepherded Ludwig Bemelmans' Madeline and her classmates two by two in a neat file around Paris.

Ingrid Betancourt, 49, a politician with dual Columbian and French citizenship is a good example of that shoulder-length hairstyle in the dark mahogany shade popular with chic French women of certain age. The waist length black hair streaked with gray braided and wrapped around her head at the time of her dramatic rescue from the jungles of Columbia where she had been held captive by the FARC group has now been trimmed. It has been given a new, rich mahogany tone that gives her olive skin a warm glow.

A photo taken recently at a talk Ingrid Betancourt made in the USA shows a beautiful smiling woman who might be the daughter of the woman whose face we saw the day of her rescue from six and a half years under difficult jungle conditions. Comparing photos of Ingrid Betancourt the day of her rescue with photos taken at the time of the launch of her book *Even Silence Has an End: My Six Years of Captivity in the Colombian Jungle* in September 2010 should convince us all of the possibilities for repairing damage when we have been through periods of great stress and could not give face and body proper care.

Another chic French woman who chooses the shoulder length mahogany hair is Fadéla Amara, 46, a French feminist and human rights advocate. Born in France to Algerian immigrant parents in a poor suburb, she is currently the French Secretary of State for urban regeneration. Her thick fringe of bangs bring attention to Fadéla Amara's deep brown eyes. In her campaign for rights of women, Fadéla Amara is extremely vocal in her opposition to the burka, the body covering and veil she calls a prison and a straight jacket for women. And a burka certainly makes it impossible to see a chic French hairstyle.

French actress Sophie Duez, 48, also often wears her long, dark brown hair cut with a thick fringe of bangs. A native of Nice on the French Riviera she has recently been a member of the Nice city council and has now taken the position of responsibility for converting the old abattoirs into artists workshops. Sophie Duez told an interviewer for *Madame Figaro* that she maintains her hair with *Masque Fleur de Jasmine* and the *Shampooing au Miel* by Leonor Greyl, Paris. These pricey natural hair products are the choice of a number of chic French women whose lifestyle demands beautiful, luxurious hair.

Presidential candidate Segolène Royal, 57, is yet one more example of the shoulder length mahogany hair certain age choice. During the campaign she was observed maintaining her style with frequent brushing. Brushing might seem old-fashioned, but for many women it is a simple, economical way to keep certain age hair healthy and shiny. Certain age hair also benefits from avoiding overly hot water for shampooing that would strip out natural oils. Finishing, as French women do, with a final cold water rinse to help seal in those natural oils and any conditioners you might have used also helps.

But what is that very distinct mahogany hair color so popular with French women of a certain age?

Commercial products are used, as certainly they are in the case of the celebrity clients of color guru Christophe Robin. But for many French women that mahogany shade, done in a salon or as a DIY home project, is henna.

Henna is a natural plant product that has been used for centuries as a hair treatment and body decoration in many countries around the world. So popular today in France, henna is imported by the ton! Hundreds of thousands of pounds of the powder every year.

Henna's appeal to French women is that it fits their preference for natural botanical products for skin and hair care. Products we put directly on skin and hair are absorbed into our bodies. Chic French women believe the botanical products are safer and healthier. Ecological factors figure too. Chemical hair color products put chemicals in our waste systems that municipal treatment systems can't always successfully remove. In some areas there are no treatment systems. Water discharged from households and salons goes directly into waterways. Henna is natural and poses no problems for the environment.

Also, since most French women elect to keep there natural hair color when defining their personal style, henna is an easy next step when gray begins to appear. Henna is permanent. When a woman's amount of gray is still at a minimum, henna can be applied once and touch-ups done when needed at the part and hairline.

Warning: Henna should not be applied to hair that has been bleached or processed with any chemical hair color. To do so risks a really weird hair color, or worse, damaged hair that breaks off at the roots. Nor can you safely put chemical hair color on hair that has been hennaed.

Today henna is not much used for hair color in the USA. But once Americans loved henna. Or at least they loved a women who created her red hair with henna. Lucille Ball, the comedienne who starred in the television series *I Love Lucy* had a so-so acting career with her natural dark hair. But as her daughter Lucy Arnaz has explained, once Lucy went red, it unlocked a comedy genius that made Lucille Ball one of the most successful and best-loved comedians of the 20th century. A good lesson here in the importance of finding the right hair color for your personality. You may not be born with it, but you can certainly create it.

French women's preference for shades of color with very warm red tones makes a statement about their approach to aging, I think. Lucia Mace, the stylist responsible for the red locks of "Mad Men's" Joan Holloway character told *The New York Times*: "Out of all the colors [red] makes the most statement — it infers personality. Red is wild and sexy and powerful." Those red highlights in chic French women's hair perhaps are there to make the statement that they have no intention of fading quietly into old age.

While Americans were watching *I Love Lucy* in the 1950s, they were also viewing a lot of advertising in the media for hair color products designed to make the practice more acceptable to "nice" woman by removing the taint of hair color as something done by women of questionable morals. Advertising campaigns in the USA also convinced American women that they would have more fun and look more attractive as blondes. Today, it is hard to pin down precisely what percentage of American women use a hair color product on their hair. You can see figures from 51 to 75 percent. But in the USA, the majority of women who use hair color products choose blond shades, whether created by changing the color of all the hair or by highlighting.

Not so with chic French women, blondes are still in the minority. And according to information in *Marie-Claire*, French women who go for lighter shades want subtle highlights over their natural base. Spending more money on hair color annually than women in other European countries, French women prefer their highlights painted on in a process called *balayage*. This process gives more natural highlights with the advantage of longer time between touch-ups than foiled or capped highlights. Many of the chic women discussed in these pages who choose brown shades can be seen with highlighting.

One whose rich brown hair can be seen with highlighting is French actress, now also film director, Fanny Ardant, 62. She has maintained her rich dark hair throughout her career generally at mid-length and with a free, very feminine tousle of curls that also gives her a youthful look

If the interviewer describes a woman in her mid-70s skin as "glowing," it is a good sign that hair color is harmonious with skin tone. That hair color is dark brown for French actress Leslie Caron, 79, busy with her film roles and supervising her *Auberge la Lucarne aux Chouettes* about 80 miles southeast of Paris. *Los Angeles Times* travel writer Susan Spano on a visit to the *auberge* in 2006 when Leslie Caron was 75, described her: "a petite woman with dark brown hair, over 60, I guessed, but how much older I couldn't say because she had beautiful skin, luminous green eyes and a very light step."

Dark brown is also the choice of the "richest woman in Europe," L'Oréal heiress Liliane Bettencourt, 87. Her choice has special significance because it was her father Eugene Schueller who as a young French chemist developed in 1907 the first modern chemical hair color product that he sold to Parisian hairdressers. His company first called *Société Française de Teintures Inoffensives pour Cheveux* (French Society of Harmless Color for Hair) was soon renamed L'Oréal, still a world leader in hair color products. Interesting, I think, that the fortune of the "richest woman in Europe" is built on hair and skin care products.

Looking at photos or even seeing a woman face-to-face, it is not always easy to tell the difference between henna and that rich reddish brown shade created with chemical hair color. Writer Nancy Huston, 57, French by long residence, is the only one of the chic women I surveyed whose mahogany hair I am reasonably certain is hennaed. The 2007 winner of France's *Prix Femina* for her novel *Lignes de Faille* (Fault LInes) was born in Alberta, Canada. In

1973 she went to Paris for her junior year abroad. Paris has been her home since that time. In her essay on being beautiful, "Dealing With What's Dealt" written shortly after her 40th birthday, Nancy Huston tells her readers that she has begun putting henna on her shoulder length hair to cover the gray.

Another writer who chooses shoulder length hair is Calixthe Beyala, 49. For her style, it is a profusion of thick, ebony-hued natural curls that frame her smooth, dark, often-smiling face. Calixthe Beyala is about as close as France comes to having an Oprah—with a dash of Jane Fonda at her politically active phase. A chief difference, however, between the French and American women is that Calixthe Beyala is a writer of books who makes frequent media appearances. Oprah Winfrey is a media figure who has promoted the sale of millions of books by her recommendations.

Though Calixthe Beyala was born in Cameroon, West Africa, coming to France in her late teens, Sylvie Genevoix, writing for *Madame Figaro*, describes this most successful female writer from Francophone Africa as *"Parisienne jusqu'au bout des ongles."* Parisienne to the tips of her toes. Calixthe Beyala is both highly commercially successful and the winner of literary awards including the *Grand Prix du roman de l'Académie Française*. She has also provoked controversy, in part for her campaigning for the inclusion of more actors of African heritage in French cinema.

Another writer with African heritage, Marie NDiaye, 43, chooses to crop short her curly black hair. Winner of France's most prestigious literary prize, the Goncourt (previous winners include Marcel Proust and Simone de Beauvoir), for her novel *Trois Femmes Puissantes* (Three Strong Women), the writer was born in France to a French mother and a Senegalese father. Marie NDiaye shares with President Barack Obama that her African father left when she was too young to remember him and she did not see him again until many years later. Like Calixthe Beyala, she is inclined to political statements. When Nicholas Sarkozy was elected president of France, Marie NDiaye declared Sarkozy, among other things: *"vulgaire."* She packed up and moved to Berlin apparently for the remainder of Sarkozy's term in office.

Writer Françoise Bourdin, 58, also favors very short hair. Her style choice is a neat, silvering cap with side part and sweep of bangs across her forehead. For a prolific novelist and screenwriter who is also an accomplished horsewoman, it is a flattering and practical hairstyle. Françoise Bourdin, whose books include *D'espoir et de promessee* (Of Hope & Promise), *Sans regrets* (Without Regrets) and *Dans le silence de l'aube* (In the Silence of the Dawn) assures prospective readers that her novels are "stories about people like us." Given that much current French fiction seems populated by any number of troubled, sociopathic characters, "like us" is very reassuring.

French painter and writer Françoise Gilot, 89, has lived the certain age portion of her life in the USA. The dark shade and the length of her hair has varied through these years. But in February 2010 at the time of her show at the Mann Gallery in New Orleans her French mahogany hair was cut short in a youthful parted-on-the-left, barrette-on-the-right style. Françoise Gilot, by the way, is the mother of jewelry designer Paloma Picasso, 61, discussed previously in this section.

Kristin Scott Thomas, 50, is, of course, British. But I include her as one of the "chic French women of certain age" not only because of her long residence in France, but because her style and attitudes are so French.

In her several decades of film, we have sometimes seen the actress as a blonde as in *The English Patient*. But more often her hair has been dark brown and shoulder length. Sometimes with bangs, but more often swept back to show us that Kristin Scott Thomas forehead balanced perfectly by her wide mouth.

An Italian actress whom I believe also qualifies as one of the book's "chic French women of certain age" is Laura Morante, 54. Like Kristin Scott Thomas, she has played notable roles in numerous French films. In 2008 she was chosen to be the *ambassadrice* for the French skin care company Lancôme's Absolue line. *"Discrète et tellement belle, elle incarne idéalement la femme Absolue de Lancôme, un rôle qui lui colle à la peau."* Distinctly and truly beautiful, she is the ideal incarnation of the Absolue de Lancôme, a role that fits her like a glove, said Lancôme.

As with all actresses, Laura Morante's hair color and style is often determined by the film role in which she appears. Most often we have seen her hair in a rich dark brown shade worn up with a sweep of luxurious bangs across her forehead that sets off her dark brown eyes.

Despite the popularity of the darker shades of hair color for French certain age. Loulou de la Falaise, 62, owner of the Left Bank boutique *Maison de Loulou*, prefers a lighter hair color. Italian *Vogue* described her hairstyle in a June 2010 profile: "short, artfully messy, dark blond."

Artfully messy is favored by some chic French women in all age groups. Why don't they just comb their hair? some Americans ask. Because for many face shapes, artfully messy is a more flattering frame for the face, especially a small face on a woman who has fine hair. And artfully messy is sexy. In Loulou de la Falaise's case, one would not expect someone who was expelled from three boarding schools and was part of the Studio 54 crowd in its heyday to wear her hair tamed back into a neat little gray bun.

Loulou de la Falaise is often tagged as Yves Saint Laurent's muse. She is quick to point out, however, that in her 30 years with that design house, she did not sit around looking prettily inspirational. She put in long hours of very hard work.

Writer Madeleine Chapsal, 85, wears her fiery red hair in a shoulder length frizz. No gray locks for this lively octogenarian who is still penning one, sometimes two, three or four books a year. Her latest publication in 2010 was *A qui tu pense quand tu me fais l'amour?* Who Are You Thinking Of When You Make Love To Me? This is not the sort of title usually found on books written by women in their mid-80s. Certainly not in the USA. Like those of the 20th century French writer Colette (who also chose frizzy red hair in certain age) Madeleine Chapsal's books have a large audience with women because she writes from a personal viewpoint about issues important in their lives. One of her books published in 2006 was *Le certain âge*.

For a distinctive, not like other chic French women of certain age hairstyle, the prize surely should go to Carine Roitfeld, 56, for ten years the editor-in-chief of French *Vogue*, who in December 2010 announced her decision to leave the magazine. Her long, straight, honey-brown, parted-in-the-middle hair reaches the middle of her back. Frequently hair on one side falls down over one eye in sort of a hippie chick meets 1940s glamor girl effect. Whether one eye or two are visible, her eyes are thickly lined in dark black kohl beneath her strong, dark brows. A number of journalists have pointed out a resemblance of Carine Roitfeld to the singer Iggy Pop. I do not think this is meant as a compliment. Still the effect of the lanky hair and starkly dark eyes and her often black outfits are softened by the genuine smile she wears. The ultra-thin fashionista in her impossibly high designer heels and her surprising combinations of couture styles is considered the height of Paris chic by her devoted admirers around the world. In photos often taken by The Sartorialist and by the fashion media, Carine Roitfeld always looks chic and certainly more youthful and energetic than a great many other chic French women, like her, a few years short of 60.

Looking at color photos of Carine Roitfeld, it struck me that her hair color appeared to be very natural. Research found a Sartorialist posting that listed her Paris colorist as Romain Colors. The chicest of the Paris *bio-chic* salons *spécialisé depuis 2002 dans la coloration douce, organique, naturelle et végétale et au balayage à l'argile,* specializing since 2002 in gentle organic, natural and vegetal hair coloring, and in clay highlighting.

THE TREND IN PARIS NOW is for more environmentally-sensitive hair salons that use products less damaging to water and soil, not to mention the human bodies to which they are applied. New natural and organic hair salons are springing up all over Paris—and no doubt in other French cities as well. No less than the *Scientific American* tells us that salons, similar to those *bio-chic* French salons, are opening in many major cities across the USA. These salons use non-toxic and/or organic ingredients in interiors featuring energy efficient lighting, non-toxic insulation and low-VOC paints. The magazine suggests to find such a salon in your area, type in "green salon" and your two letter state abbreviation into an internet search engine. You might also try "organic hair salon" in your search.

My search for at-home hair color products sold in the USA that avoid environment damaging chemicals turned up three sorts of products. First were those that were pure henna and could not be used over hair that had been previously chemically colored, at least until all the chemically treated hair had grown out and been cut off. Second were products with henna and chemicals combined. And third were products that advertised natural and organic ingredients, but a reading of the labels found almost as many—and many of the same chemicals—as in commercial hair color products. The prices for these "natural" hair color products were higher, sometimes more than double, the price of chemical hair color products.

When it comes to chic certain age haircuts, perhaps French women are at some advantage. They live in a country where hair is very important and many talented people are drawn to the profession. Also many French women have the type of natural curl in their hair that they can stand in front of a mirror with nail scissors and snip away at their hair, and when they are finished, they look as if they enjoyed the services of a top stylist.

Life is not fair.

But these days you can have a reasonably chic haircut almost everywhere. You may have to search a bit for the right stylist. If your search finds nothing promising, you may need to find a stylist looking to build a clientele who will be willing to work with you to cut the style you want.

As for hair color, if you aren't satisfied with the work at salons in your area, or if you don't like their prices, home hair color products are better than ever. A wealth of good how-to information is available online. For instance, Christophe Robin, the Paris colorist I quoted who takes care of all those chic celebrities, is also the technical guru for L'Oréal Paris' popular Preference hair-color. You can access his home hair color advice on the L'Oréal website.

I BEGAN *CHIC & SLIM TOUJOURS* WITH HAIR, not only because I employ the top-to-toe format, I also used this hair section to introduce you to some chic French women who offer us style and lifestyle inspiration. You will learn more about many of them in future sections. Most important I began with hair because a chic French woman's hairstyle is important to her, and because decisions about your hair are fundamental choices you will make in designing your certain age personal style. Robin Givhan writing on hair for women of certain age in the *Washington Post* said:

> Hair tells a story as well, but its tales are especially personal — more intimate than clothes could ever be. Hair speaks about politics, culture, social standing and even religion. But it also speaks to our race, ethnicity and health. We treat our hair like precious treasure. Women are particularly disinclined to trust just anyone with it. They will follow a beloved hairstylist hither and yon rather than attempt to build a relationship with someone new. The decision to cover gray strands — or not — can tap into self-confidence and the way in which they will engage with the world.

Chic French women of certain age engage the world with great self-confidence. Their personal style announces that confidence beginning with their choice of hairstyle and color. They make that choice after careful thought. You should give your certain age hairstyle and color choice careful thought as well.

LETTERS TO ANNE BARONE
About *Chic & Slim*

Thank you for remaining so faithful to American women. We need your techniques now more than ever.
Crystal

Just a note to say THANK YOU for all that you have done and for all you continue to do to create happy, healthy, chic women (and consequently their families) across the country. You are one in a million and I a so grateful to have found you! Your lovely, encouraging voice has made such a difference in my life.
Susan

Face

LATELY I SEE WOMEN, well-dressed, makeup-perfect women that I suspect belong to an organization called The Sisterhood of Marble Goddess Faces. So protected from the sun's rays by high SPF sunscreen, so peeled and/or lifted, so immobilized by generous amounts of Botox, so smoothed by fillers, they are beautifully, flawlessly perfect. They don't look quite real. But they do look beautiful. Just like sculptured marble goddesses.

Today we have many wonderful products and techniques for diminishing or erasing signs of age. Given that the USA is the country where "too much is never enough," not surprising many women have extensive alteration done. In the USA, both youth and money are highly respected. A woman of certain age medically edited to look younger than her daughter not only gets points for youthful appearance but also demonstrates she has the money for expensive cosmetic services.

When I was debating how to describe the American women who had extensive cosmetic alteration, I came upon a series of books written for American cosmetic dermatologists. On the cover of each book in the series is an image of the head, shoulders and décolletage of a white marble goddess with all parts flawlessly perfect. Here was the standard that American cosmetic physicians are being directed to correct American women: Marble Goddesses.

Chic French women are not so inclined toward radical improvement that would erase all imperfections. Nor for improvements that are obvious. True, esthetic anti-age treatments are on the rise in France, but the results chic French women desire are subtle. A chic French woman does not want to look younger than her daughter. She wants to look like a splendid whatever age she is. And she wants to look like herself. French doctors are happy to oblige these wishes. French rejuvenation expert Dr. George Roman who has offices in London as well as Paris was quoted in the *Daily Mail*: "In the U.S., they subscribe to one particular beauty aesthetic, so everyone ends up looking very similar." A practice he labels ridiculous. "We're human beings with different characters, physically and emotionally." He adds, "I enhance the charm of each patient, but I don't go too far, as the result has to be invisible to be successful."

I can just hear some rich Dallas woman of a certain age saying, "Well, if I pay all that money to be fixed up, I darn sure don't want the results to be *invisible!*"

But French women agree with Dr. Roman's philosophy. They think that the extent of work many American women choose produces a faux, unnatural youthfulness that indicates desperation and discomfort with themselves. Chic French women are famously *"bien dans sa peau"* comfortable in their skin, comfortable with their appearance. Chic French women are rarely desperate.

In any case, French women (fortunate for them) are not under the same pressures as American women to erase the lines and sags from their faces when they reach certain age. In France a woman no longer young is valued for her experience. She doesn't have to look decades years younger than her biological age. She just needs to look attractive.

Chic French women don't worry so much when a few *"rides,"*

wrinkles, begin to appear on their faces, as long as they can maintain a glowing, tight-pored complexion and a svelte body. For the face, that means facials, and peels, and a well-stocked supply of skin care products that would include (among others) cleansing milks or creams or a specialty soap, toners, moisturizers, anti-redness creams, eye creams, nourishing oils, day creams, night replenishing lotions, masques, and lip balms. The same types of skin care products used by American women.

What brands of skin care do French women use? I have often been asked. Actually many of the same brands women all over the world use. After all, Clarins, Yves Rocher, Lancôme and L'Oréal, and numerous others popular in the USA are French companies. French stores stock many brands made outside France, certainly many skin care lines made in the USA. For instance, in October 2010, *Sephora* France listed its best-selling skin care product for the face was the American company's Estée Lauder's Advanced Night Repair Concentrate. *Les soins anti-âge* are hot sellers in France in all brands.

Yet keep in mind that what is bestselling online at *Sephora* France might not be the bestseller in the country. Many other websites sell skin care. Neighborhood pharmacies sells skin care products. As do *supermarchés* and department stores. Some skin care brands have their own stores. Many estheticians and pharmacists sell their own or favorite brands. In her 2009 autobiography *Thank Heaven*, the French actress Leslie Caron tells readers that when she was a child, her father, a chemist, created his own line of beauty products that he sold in his Paris *pharmacie*.

Like the trend in hair care, the current trend in French skin care is for more natural and less synthetic and chemical ingredients. Many chic French women are now choosing *les produits de beauté naturel et cosmétiques bio*, natural and organic skin care and makeup. These items are sold in specialty stores and specialty websites as well as from the stores and websites of the companies making these *naturel* and *bio* products. They are also sold in the new Naturalia stores, a French chain selling a product range much like our Whole Foods. Toward the end of this section I have more to say about this *naturel et bio* trend. And about some of these skin care products popular with chic French women.

Like women all over the world, chic French women today make skin care product choices from reading magazine and online reviews, from blogs and websites, from recommendations from their esthetician or dermatologist, and by keeping an eye out for what other chic women are using.

Chic French women budget for skin care products and treatments as necessities. Ten percent of income is a figure often quoted. While in the past French women might choose one brand of skin care and cosmetics and use the products of that brand exclusively, this no longer seems to be the case. And while in the past French women might choose a product and remain devoted to that product for years, concern about the health hazards of some ingredients in some skin care and makeup products are causing many to switch to products certified natural and organic by recognized certifying organizations such as EcoCert and Cosmébio. Another reason for switching is because recently new products have appeared that offer dramatically more effective treatments, especially for women of certain age. For instance, some of these new rub-on hyaluronic acid products offer a quick, if temporary, erasure of those certain age wrinkles without injections of the filler.

Michèle Fitoussi, 56, has been an editor at French *Elle* for over 25 years. One of her earlier non-fiction books was an Oprah Club selection. Her book *Superwoman's had enough* was a bestseller in France. Her latest book is *Helena Rubinstein, la femme qui inventa la beauté*. In a French *Vogue* interview about the new book, Michèle

Fitoussi mentions as an aside that she uses Clinique. That Clinique, by the way, is an American skin care line, owned and developed by Estée Lauder, Helena Rubinstein's great rival. Michèle Fitoussi calls Helena Rubinstein, the woman who invented *la beauté*, as in *institut de beauté*, the French skin care salons to which chic French women are so devoted. The title rendered in English would be: the woman who invented the beauty business. In promoting her business, Helena Rubinstein also did a service for women by countering the notion that respectable women did not improve on their natural looks. The feisty little Polish-born entrepreneur convinced women that for their own sakes they could improve and preserve their beauty, a lesson particularly needed by American women living in a Puritanical society.

The Rubinstein book also links women's changing beliefs about enhancing their beauty and early women's liberation. Notable that today, societies most repressive of women's rights require them to cover themselves in various garments that prevents the viewing of even their faces and hair. In some of these societies, the simple act of having one's hair styled at a salon will earn brutal physical punishment—sometimes disfigurement. Why? Because enhancing a woman's physical attractiveness is liberating and empowering.

The corrective treatments for my face done beginning a decade ago in my mid-50s were a liberation from the restrictions that my facial defects were putting on my life.

By the time I completed the second *Chic & Slim* book, *Chic & Slim Encore*, I was close to becoming a recluse because of problems on my face. First of all there was my nose scar that every doctor who had looked at it (except one) had said that because of its type and location any surgical attempt to repair it would likely make it worse. The one doctor who said he had a new technique that would repair the scar had previously done a wonderful job removing some large, unsightly moles and left absolutely no scars. Unfortunately his attempt at nose repair did not work. I was left an uglier scar than before.

Hardly a quarter of an inch from the nose scar was a bright red spot that was increasing in size. A vein had broken one morning during an ice storm when I had walked my young son to school. I should not have been outside in those frigid temperatures because of a circulatory condition. The doctor who had diagnosed that circulatory condition in my mid-20s had said, "It won't kill you, but when you are middle-age, the veins will start breaking around your nose and everyone will think you are an alcoholic." Oh, great!

The veins around my nose did begin breaking in my early 50s, as the doctor had predicted. If the scar, the big red broken vein and the red lines radiating out both sides of my nose weren't enough, there were the acne scars covering my cheeks and chin. Either I would have some work done or really become a recluse.

Fortunately, lasers for dealing with unsightly veins had been developed. A local esthetic physician was reported to do good work. I made an appointment for a laser treatment. You may make your appointment for broken veins on your nose, but once at the clinic, you may find, as I did, that first you are going to have to endure a lengthy sales session for the clinic's other services. You may be shown videos. You may be photographed so that you may see your many defects more clearly. You may be given demonstrations. Certainly you will be given booklets and sales brochures. Your own personal improvement program will be charted. Finally comes the punch line: For a mere $5000 to $20,000 you too can become an official member of The Sisterhood of the Marble Goddess Faces.

At this point, some women, as one of my friends did, angrily walk out of the clinic and never have any work done. At least not there. My own strategy in this instance was to play it a little cagey. "Let's just go ahead and take care of the veins today. I want some time to think about all these other services so I can decide which I might want."

When I got into the treatment room, the doctor took one look at me and rightly deduced that I wasn't a likely candidate for those more pricey Sisterhood services and upped the price the sales rep had quoted 50 percent. I readily agreed. I wanted those unsightly red veins off my nose, and I was perfectly willing to pay what the doctor believed his services were worth. Besides, the doctor's gruff, almost-hostile manner did not invite discussion. (I later was told his manner was related to his health. He died a few weeks after he did my work.)

Despite his health problems, his laser work was excellent. The red lines radiating out from the side of my nose were gone almost by the time I drove home from the clinic. The broken vein on top my nose took about six weeks to fade. But there were still the acne scars to deal with.

I had always avoided dermabrasion, that older, harsh grinding off of the scarred layers of skin. A friend who had it done in the late 1960s had given me a scary description of how, for many painful days, her face had looked like raw hamburger. True, the dermabrasion had smoothed her acne scars, but it had left her entire face with hyperpigmentation scaring, brown spots all over her face, that I did not think was much improvement over the pits on my cheeks.

The newer microdermabrasion had no "hamburger" stage. In fact, like me, many patients look better immediately after a treatment than before because there is often a slight swelling and reddening that smooths wrinkles, makes large pores less obvious and provides a nice glow. I found an experienced technician, and in five microderm treatments spaced four weeks apart, the facial sandblasting done with wands shooting little grains against the skin erased the worst of my acne scarring.

I did have an additional five sessions that further erased scarring and smoothed the edges of my nose scar. The microderm treatments also erased those fine lines and softened those creases that had begun to appear on my mid-50s face. My skin care products began to achieve better results since part of that outer barrier of dead skin had been substantially reduced in thickness. For about $1000, I had a much improved face with side benefits.

In France, my problems that microdermabrasion treated would more likely have been taken care of with *le peeling*, chemical peels. Microderm is not done much in France. Dallas cosmetologist and spa owner Renee Rouleau, who despite her French name is Texan, explains that many French estheticians believe that microderm is too harsh and prefer to use peels. Her experience and conversations with estheticians in France have prompted her to no longer offer microderm to her clients.

Peels offered in France seem to be much the same as those offered by estheticians and dermatologists in the USA. As in America, chic French women make their choice based on the outcome they desire, their budget and how much time they have for recovery. The deepest of peels, a phenol peel, can require months of recovery and much special care. Even with a light AHA peel that requires nothing more than a good moisturizer and sun protection, those couple of days when your face, chin to forehead, is ruffled with dead skin is not the time for a big party or important business meeting.

Peels have uses beyond cosmetic. Medically, they are also being used to treat pre-cancerous growths, those pesky little bumps that seem to sprout when one reaches certain age. For

French women this means that a portion of a chemical peel might be covered by their national health insurance, just as a spa stay might be covered up to 65% for the treatment of acne.

Daphne Thioly-Bensoussan is a French dermatologist whose offices are located not far off Paris' *Champs Élysées*. Her photo accompanied an interview about chemical peels she gave to French *Elle* in October 2010. In the photo you see an excellent example of a chic French woman of certain age. Her hair which falls to the shoulders of her Mandarin-collared white doctor's uniform jacket is that dark mahogany shade so loved by French women of a certain age. Her face shows pale, but decided freckles. Beneath her well-formed brows, lines radiate out from the corners of her smiling brown eyes. She wears moderate-sized hoop earrings. Her lip stain is soft and does not detract from her eyes which have some careful lining and mascara. On her neck you can see a couple of shallow horizontal creases, normal to certain age women. But her skin glows with natural healthiness. She looks animated and fun. Men would surely find her very attractive. Her age? Who knows? Who cares?

When I checked the welcome page of Dr. Thioly-Bensoussan's website, I found, not the image of a marble goddess as those covers of the American series of cosmetic dermatology books, but a woman rendered in a colorful mosaic. Her hair is that highlighted deep rich brown so common to chic French women and her brown eyes smile and sparkle like Dr. Thioly-Bensoussan's in the *Elle* photo. Her skin is not marble white, but her olive-toned skin is sun-kissed with healthy color on her cheeks, chin, forehead and nose. Her earrings add decoration to her attractive face. She looks content. Still, she is not perfect. There on her forehead, and again on her lip, and in two places on her neck a small piece of the mosaic is missing. She shows some age. But she is still very beautiful. Very approachable.

If the perfect marble statue with its flawless, immobile face, unaffected by any ray of sun is the model which American women want their cosmetic treatments, the beautiful woman in Dr. Thioly-Bensoussan's website welcome mosaic is the model which chic French women prefer.

Jeanine Dumaret, a French esthetic physician who is *specialiste des interventions anti-âge*, pointed out in a French *Vogue* article that the human face has 52 points of aging. To rejuvenate a face, all those 52 points must be taken into account so that the treatment will balance the face. The healing phase must be carefully managed. Otherwise the results will not be natural. Chic French women want natural.

Despite all those Marble Goddess faces we see, many American women want natural-looking results in esthetic interventions. One of my friends at 60 had a slim, trim body of which any 25-year-old would be envious. But she had inherited genes for washboard facial wrinkling that no skin care product had been able to ameliorate. Her face, unfortunately, looked 20 years older than her actual age. After a careful consultation, a cosmetic surgeon designed a combination of surgery and Botox that gave her a face more in line with her actual age. The result was extremely natural and she felt comfortable with the change.

My friend's work was done several years ago. Now in place of Botox, the doctor might use one of the hyaluronic acid fillers such as Restylane or Juvéderm. These fillers are increasingly chosen by esthetic physicians and their patients because they do not interfere with facial movement. They are widely offered in France as they are in the USA.

Botox remains very popular here in the USA. Since I am still squeamish about have the world's deadliest toxin injected into my body, I am still quite happy using Frownies. These little pieces of adhesive-backed brown paper that you stick on various points of the face to retrain the muscle do the job that Botox is designed to do. Frownies have been around for more than a 100 years. You can buy a lifetime supply for about the cost of one treatment of Botox. But Frownies do have disadvantages. First, you have to wear them at least three hours a day to get results. And you do look odd with that brown paper stuck here and there on your face.

IF AMERICAN WOMEN HAVE NEVER as firmly embraced French women's habit of regular facials done by a professional esthetician at a skin care salon, it is surely due in part to better American bathrooms.

From the time most American middle-class housing became equipped with indoor plumbing, bathrooms in the USA have been oases of luxury compared to French bathrooms. An American woman could assemble her skin care products and settle in for a relaxing weekly or monthly facial in the comfort and privacy of her home. Women's magazines, women's sections of newspapers, and books by skin care specialists provided plenty of at-home, how-to instructions. An American woman could find most of the ingredients needed for an at-home facial in her kitchen or bathroom, or she could buy them at her neighborhood drug store or department store cosmetic counter.

Christine Valmy was a Romanian-born skin care specialist who immigrated to the USA in 1961 and established salons and a school of esthetics. In *Christine Valmy's Skin Care and Makeup Book* (1982) the ingredients required for her at-home facial for dry skin listed the daytime moisturizer and night cream a woman regularly used, grated cucumber, raw oatmeal, hops extract, ginseng tea, wheat germ oil, mashed peaches and cotton balls. Though I would point out, that Christine Valmy's skin care, still in business today, has moved beyond grated cucumber and mashed peaches for at-home facials. The company sells a Gold Collagen anti-aging masque that contains 24 karat gold-flakes in addition to gotu kola, bilberry and echinacea.

What skin care salons existed in the USA in the 20th century were usually in larger cities and often run by foreign-born and foreign-trained skin care specialists, many French. In any case, for skin problems not responding to home care, an American woman was likely to see her family doctor or a dermatologist rather than an esthetician.

Today an increasing number of American women are having facials, peels and other esthetic procedures at skin care salons in every city of any size and even in many small towns. At the same time, more French women are seeing a dermatologist for their skin care. Not only is a dermatologist's treatment more likely to be covered, at least in part, under the national health insurance, but French cosmetic dermatologists can offer stronger treatments with better results than an esthetician. The same is true in the USA. Though here we have an in-between type of institution, a medi-spa, technically a medical spa, a physician-directed salon that offers the regular salon/spa type treatments such as facials and massages, but also offers the medical anti-age treatments including Botox and hyaluronic fillers, and a number of the machine esthetic procedures such as Endermologie or photo facials. These are generally performed by a technician or registered nurse rather than the doctor.

At the medi-spa, where I was having my microderm, their Botox and hyaluronic acid filler injections were given by a RN. A friend having her first experience with Botox went to a doctor, actually a cosmetic surgeon who had long experience not only with facelifts and such, but the other popular esthetic procedures as well. With 21 tiny injections he sculpted her face so that in one session 20 years were erased. I saw her both shortly before and after her Botox and had known her 20 years previously. Amazing.

But Botox wears off in about four months and to maintain the correction, more Botox is needed. Rather than drive the distance to the doctor who had done the first Botox and pay his higher price, she made an appointment at the medi-spa. I knew their system of Botox was one injection in the forehead frown lines. I warned my friend that she would not be as happy with the medi-spa's Botox injection as she had been with the doctor's treatment. She wasn't.

Having one's work done by a dermatologist might save money in the long run. Before I had laser epilation to treat the part of my facial hair that my six years of electrolysis in the 1980s had not eliminated, I did extensive research on laser hair removal. Nowhere at that time did I encounter the information that for five percent of patients laser hair removal will not work because of hormonal problems. (I actually found the information in the patient information on the website of the Paris cosmetic dermatologist Daphne Thioly-Bensoussan while researching this book.) The day I kept my appointment at my local medi-spa for my first laser treatment for facial hair, I was given a multi-page legal document to sign that can be summarized: *This probably won't work, but you are going to have to pay for it anyway.* It didn't work. I had to pay for it anyway.

At least in France, screening by a dermatologist who gives laser epilation treatments would likely have identified me as not a good candidate because my facial hair was the result of hormonal problems. I would have saved money. My five treatments at the medi-spa were $100 each.

Even though many chic French women are choosing to have their peels and other cosmetic procedures done by cosmetic dermatologists, French women still patronize their *instituts de beauté*. Americans got a good look at a typical *institut* in the 1999 film *Venus Beauté*, the film that introduced French actress Audrey Tautou in a supporting role. My pleasure in the film was increased because I viewed the DVD version while I was in the midst of my treatments at skin care salons here in North Texas. I saw similarities, particularly in the type of treatments offered.

Instituts de beauté in France offer the facials, peels, permanent makeup, massages, waxing, manicures, pedicures, cellulite therapy, laser hair removal, teeth whitening, tattoo removal, Botox, hyaluronic fillers and skin care products that you find in many skin care salons in cities across the USA. You can have the French Bio Visage facial using noninvasive microcurrent and 40 botanicals and extracts at an *institut de beauté* in France, but also at many salons and medi-spas in the USA. Cellulite therapies such as Cellu M6 are available in France as in the USA.

Something relatively new on the beauty scene in France are chains of *instituts de beauté* that offer low cost, no frills services to customers on a subscription basis. The French chains will also serve those who do not have a subscription/membership, but those customers pay a higher price for treatments. Ingrid Haberfeld checked out the service at two of these chains for *France Soir*. She was pleased with the quality of the leg waxing at Espace Épilation and with the facial masque at Body Minute. The pampering in relaxing and decorative ambiance common to most beauty institutes was missing, however.

Treatment areas in both low-cost institutes were small. Sound passed through thin partitions between treatment areas. But in a tough economy, prices were good: 6.5€ (about $9) for the half-leg waxing and 35€ (about $47) for the facial. Compare to prices at traditional *instituts*: 75€ ($100) for a facial, 100€ ($133) for a body treatment and 50€ ($67) for leg waxing. In a tough economy, these low-cost institutes make it possible for French women on a tight budget to have beauty services they might not otherwise be able to afford. The verdict: *Des soins de qualités mais sans chichi.* Quality beauty treatments, but without frills.

At the next level of beauty services, a cosmetic dermatologist in a major city in France will offer much the same services as one in a major city in the USA: surely treating acne and skin cancers, but esthetic procedures as well. Many are the same as in a salon or medi-spa: Botox, cellulite therapies, laser facial treatments, skin resurfacing and hair removal, liposuction, photo facials, pigment and tattoo removal. But the cosmetic dermatologist likely would also offer other physician services such as stronger peels, sclerotherapy for veins, mole removal, facial vein elimination, eyelid rejuvenation, ear lobe repair, and treatment of rosacea.

Clinics that provide cosmetic surgeries in the two countries also offer similar services. They will redo your nose, rejuvenate your face, augment your breasts with traditional surgery. Their laser surgeries can renew your skin and remove unwanted hair. At the same time you can have hair restored to places it is wanted, varicose veins treated, photo facials, Botox, and fillers. At these clinics, doctors can remove your freckles, your age spots and the fat on your thighs.

In both France and the USA, often these clinics, in order to provide a certain discretion for their patients, are located in smaller cities. For instance the *Clinique Saint-Aubin, spécialiste de la médecine anti-âge* is in Toulouse, a city in the south of France where unless someone had great interest in historic architecture, really good cassoulet, or the Airbus factory, they might be unlikely to visit. Though Toulouse is in the region just east of Provence and the French Riviera. Likewise, Abilene on the windy Texas plains has established itself as a cosmetic surgery center, 150 miles west of Dallas. Distant enough for discretion, but close enough for convenience.

In both France and the USA, the chic, but budget-minded, sometimes seek treatment outside their own country. When I lived in South Texas in the 1990s, word was that you could go to Monterrey, Mexico, and have "20 years taken off for $4000." The work was reported to be excellent. Now, of course, because of threat of violence from drug wars raging in the US-Mexico border area, you might get excellent esthetic treatment, but you might also find transport home in a hand-carved Mexican coffin. Alas.

While treatments offered in the USA and France might be much the same, the experience at an American or a French facility might be very different. From my experience, and from complaints voiced by others, in the USA, one's pleasure is sometimes marred by the hard sell for other products and services often by pointing out, not particularly tactfully, your many areas needing improvement. Supposedly a facial, a massage, or peel is to be stress-relieving and pampering. But if another employee is constantly barging into the treatment room hunting some supply or delivering a phone message, this can spoil the ambience. I have had root canals that left me more relaxed and de-stressed than some of my supposed-to-be-relaxing medi-spa sessions here in North Texas.

France has a long tradition of skin care and beauty maintenance, seen, not as a luxury, but a necessity for French women. Perhaps for this reason, the standards for training and certification are much higher in France than the USA. Any esthetician in France will have had lengthy training and passed a rigorous two-day exam. Many working as estheticians in the USA have been trained and certified as hairdressers, but beyond that they may only have been given a little how-to knowledge from other estheticians or doctors for whom they work in a medi-spa.

Many products and devices used in esthetic skin and body treatments were developed in France and were in use there before they were introduced in the USA. For these and other factors, you are more likely to get more expert treatment in France than in the USA. Though, if you are selective, you can get excellent treatment in the USA. If your personal style is closer to chic French than chic American, however, you may have difficulty in getting the results you want. *Thank you, but I really don't want to join the Sisterhood of the Marble Goddess Faces.*

HOW MANY CHIC FRENCH WOMEN are having esthetic anti-aging treatments beyond basic skin care facials, light peels and the salon facial massages? Impossible to say since French women and their doctors prefer subtle results and since French women are reticent to admit these treatments. Despite all the new skin care products and high-tech treatments available, French women, with their strong preference for the simple and natural, are reportedly remaining impressively faithful to traditional home skin care routines.

The French nightly routine has long been a quick cleansing with a *lait de toilette*, cleansing milk, at bedtime. These cleansing milks have the convenience that they are applied and removed with a cotton ball or pad. No rinsing with water needed, but a follow up with a *tonique*, toner is often recommended.

Three sorts of *laits de toilette* are popular. Some labeled *bébé*, are for cleaning baby's skin, others (sometimes labeled *lait demaquillant*, makeup remover) are designated adult cosmetic use. Yet other *laits de toilette* are sold as suitable for baby's tender bottom, as well as mama's or grandmama's pretty face. High in botanicals, many brands are *bio*, organic. Most are low in, or without chemicals. These *laits de toilette* nourish as well as cleanse.

Since so many French women have that fair, tight-pored, Northern European skin not inclined to producing dirt-trapping excessive oil that plague women of other ethnic heritages, this system apparently works satisfactorily. And since many French women do not wear foundation makeup, its removal at nighttime is not a factor. Though most of these *laits de toilette* are formulated for dry or sensitive skin. Oilier skin or faces that need to remove makeup often require stronger products. These also are applied with a cotton pad. Some require rinsing with water, others need following with an herbal toner to complete the cleansing.

I have always been envious of French women's traditional morning skin cleansing routine: a splash of water on the face. Preferably patted dry with a white cotton piqué towel or other lint free fabric. (Turkish toweling can leave little fibers on the face.) How simple! How quick! Tap water might be used, but since much water in France is "hard" and thus drying, a bottled mineral water with a fairly neutral ph is preferred. Evian, also much used to mix with infant formula, is popular for the morning toilette.

The actress Laura Morante told French *Elle* in an interview for their *Beauté des stars* feature that her morning beauty routine was a spray with either Evian or Avène mineral water followed by a *tonique* (toner). Following the mineral water spray she applies only a *crème de jour*, day cream.

Several years ago, I read an interview with a French actress (Juliette Binoche, I think) in which when asked about a beauty routine, mentioned the morning splash of water. Wonderful if that is all your skin needs. Unfortunately, if your skin is oily or inclined to breakouts, water only in the morning will not suffice. I tried it once for three days. Oh dear! Breakouts! Some of us need a good cleanser night and morning.

ONE COMPANY THAT MAKES CLEANSERS popular with chic French women that has come to the forefront of the natural and organic skin care trend is *Laboratoires Cattier*. (Not be confused with that other French company named Cattier that produces Champagne.) For 40 years *Laboratoires Cattier* have been making France's bestselling natural products for babies. Today those mamas who came to love Cattier for their children can buy products to pamper their own skin now that they are reaching certain age.

In 2007, Cattier's *Secret Botanique*, a day cream for dry and sensitive skin, won the People's Choice Award in France for Beauty Product of the Year. Cattier's white clay facial scrub is popular with chic French women and helps make the company France's bestselling brand in the *bio* category. The white clay scrub infused with peppermint and lavender gives the face a gentle exfoliation that smooths the skin and refreshes the user.

When the magazine *60 millions de consommateurs*, 60 Million Consumers, recently tested anti-age creams on 200 women aged 40 to 65, only two *bio* anti-age creams produced results as good as regular cosmetics. One was Cattier's Nectar Eternal Anti-Âge Anti-Wrinkle Treatment. The other *bio* anti-age product that could compete with regular cosmetics was Sanoflore's *L'Elixir Anti-Âge*. Sanoflore, one of the pioneers in French organic products is now owned by L'Oréal, and as far as I have been able to learn does not have distribution in the USA. At this writing, Cattier does have distribution in USA via a website *Beautorium.com*, where you find information in English about Cattier and other *bio* products.

Just for the record, according to *France Soir*, the winner in that 60 Million Consumer test was Dior's Capture R60/80 XP with a score of 15/20. Next was a supermarket house brand product tying with L'Oréal's Anti-Wrinkle & Firming Face & Neck Moisturizer at a score of 14/20. The Dior product costs $130 for 1.7 fl. oz. L'Oréal's 1.7 fl. oz. product costs about $13 at discount stores, one-tenth the Dior cream price.

Of course chic French women who want natural and organic skin care products don't just buy those made in laboratories in France any more than they restrict themselves to regular skin care products made by French companies. Another popular *bio* brand is Weleda. The company based in Switzerland has laboratories in France as well as Germany. The good news is Weleda is widely distributed in the USA, from several websites that sell natural products, as well as at Target and Whole Foods. Weleda has a USA website in English *Usa.Weleda.com*. Weleda makes products for all types of skin, but the company's facial products for normal to oily skin based on biodynamic iris root are so popular that some won't again be available until 2011, according to the Weleda website. The luscious Wild Rose line for aging skin also has some products temporarily sold out as of this writing.

Dr. Hauschka's skin care products are also popular with chic French women. The German company founded by the Austrian chemist Rudolf Hauschka and Austrian-born esthetician Elisabeth Sigmund has been around for 40 years and has a strong presence in the USA. Dr. Hauschka skin care products are pricey—some $100 for a very small bottle. But the skin care line and its philosophy has a following worldwide. Among the American celebrities who reportedly use the products are Julia Roberts, Naomi Watts, Annette Bening, Madonna and Martha Stewart.

What is spurring this chic French move toward natural and organic skin care products?

At the most basic, the trend is simply another manifestation of the French insistence on quality. As name brand skin care products more and more contain ingredients that medical and scientific studies have shown to be harmful to humans and the environment, French are turning back to traditional beauty care ingredients. With more than 80 percent of French women employed outside the home and a population increasingly urban, this time around it's not products their *grand-mères* concocted in their kitchens from flowers and herbs grown in their gardens and collected from the hillsides. This time the natural and organic skin care cosmetics are created in laboratories by companies dedicated to quality and safety and sustainable life on the planet. Many of these companies have gardens that grow the plants from which their products are created. Those skin care products are then certified by independent organizations as to their natural and organic ingredients and that they are free from objectionable ingredients such as parabens, polyethylene glycol, phthalates, FD&C colors, sodium laurel sulfate and sodium laureth sulfate.

Two major certification organizations are Cosmébio and EcoCert. Cosmébio is the French professional association of ecological and organic cosmetics that aims to certify and thus aid consumers in identifying true natural and organic cosmetics. Makers of pseudo-*bio* products are not above plastering look-alike logos of the respected certifying organizations on their products and website product pages to give the impression of a certification they do not have. Consumers must be cautious.

EcoCert, founded in France in 1991, now inspects in more than 80 countries of the world. Inspections are primarily food and food products, but the organization also certifies textiles, detergents, perfumes, and cosmetics. The organization defines as its main objective: "To define a quality level superior to the one defined by the French and European legislation on cosmetic products, which will safeguard a real enhanced value of the natural substances used, a real practice of the respect of the environment, throughout the production process and a real respect of the consumer."

That respect for the consumer seems to be missing from many companies—numerous in the USA—that label their skin care products as organic or containing natural ingredients, but when you read the ingredient list on the label you find the product contains the same chemicals and irritating ingredients in many regular cosmetics with just a drop or two of organic flower or herbal extracts thrown in. Unfortunately, we do not have equally strong certifying organizations in the USA as in France. In the USA, there is a Natural Products Association that has been in operation since 1936. But its green and white logo is not one that I recognize or remember ever seeing on a product. For that matter I had never heard of the organization until I discovered its existence during the writing this book. In France, however, EcoCert and CosméBio are well-known among consumers interested in *bio*.

For me, our US Department of Agriculture organic certification is meaningless given how understaffed for inspections the department is and how hamstrung by industry-friendly regulations that make it impossible in many cases to adequately protect consumers. The best approach for Made in USA natural and organic skin care is to read labels carefully and take some time to research the company that produces the product. The reputable ones have websites with extensive information about their location, history and production methods. If you do not have time to do all that research yourself, you can limit your purchases to vendors whose standards equal yours and who have done the research on the companies and their products. On the *Chic & Slim* website *annebarone.com*, you will find more up-to-date information on vendors I currently find satisfactory for my own purchases of natural and organic skin care.

ANOTHER APPROACH TO SAFER MORE NATURAL and organic skin care, and one that chic French women have long used, is to make your own natural and organic cosmetics. In Linda Dannenberg's *The Paris Way of Beauty* published in 1979, there is a recipe for a "facial lotion," actually a toner, or what the French call a *tonique*. The recipe was provided to the author by *Herbier de Provence*, a Paris boutique that sold herbs and spices. You boiled five herbs (along with three more optional) in water, cooled and strained and then added some 90 percent alcohol as a preservative and bottled it and kept the toner in the refrigerator. When I lived in Corpus Christi, I could buy the small quantities of each herbal ingredient sold in bulk at my natural foods store and easily make up a batch. Today, a quick Internet search brings up lots of recipes for all sorts of natural skin care. Many as easy as making an anti-aging toner by steeping four teaspoons of green tea in one cup of boiling distilled water and straining it. Keeps a few days in the refrigerator. Apply with a cotton ball.

Under French inspiration, I have long used natural skin care in place of several sorts of commercial products. For instance, I prefer almond oil smoothed on when the skin is still damp from bathing as a body lotion. Dickinson's Witch Hazel works as a toner, though I use other toners as well. 100% cocoa butter is a great body cream. Yet I can never use cocoa butter without remembering the sultry American actress Mae West known for her large bust. When asked about a firming cream, the redoubtable Mae answered, "Cocoa butter," paused two beats and added, "Rubbed in by a man's hand." Shea butter called karité in France is a super product whose value for skin care the French learned from their days as colonists in West Africa. Pure shea butter is inexpensive and its thick texture is protective and nourishing to the skin. Shea is an ingredient in many French skin and hair products.

For my oily skin, European green clay beats any commercial facial masque product I have ever tired. Except one. About a decade ago, I was given as a gift a expensive jar of facial masque that was the mineral-rich black clay product used at one of those exclusive Italian spas where as a beauty treatment they slather you head to foot in the stuff and you come out looking as rich and beautiful as when you went in.

As I mentioned earlier, the Dr. Hauschka skin care products are popular with many celebrities in the USA, but some carry high price tags. Susan West Kurz, a licensed esthetician and president of

Dr. Hauschka Skin Care, Inc, has written *Awakening Beauty the Dr. Hauschka Way* that contains many recipes for natural ingredient treatments and beauty routines for skin and body care that puts Dr. Hauschka's science to work for us at a more economical price. The last section of the book contains many recipes for dishes one can prepare, foods to eat for beauty.

Dermonutrition, eating for beauty, is receiving attention in France. The French cosmetic dermatologist Daphne Thioly-Bensoussan I mentioned earlier in this section has, along with a couple of colleagues, written a book on the topic. As far as I can learn, their book *Les Secrets De La Dermonutrition - Bien Manger Pour Être Belle*, The Secrets of Dermonutrition: Eat Well To Be Beautiful, is available only in French.

WHILE THE HUMAN AND ENVIRONMENTAL BENEFITS of natural and organic skin care products are undeniable, those eco-friendly products have one principal drawback. Many of them simply will not do the job as well as some of the best commercial products whose ingredient lists may contain chemicals, ingredients that— though technically legal—may still pose health risks, especially from the cumulative effect when one is using concurrently several products containing the ingredient.

When I read the results of that *60 Million Consumers* test that found the Dior anti-aging cream top pick, I was not surprised. Several years ago, I received as a gift a box of Dior products. All were wonderful. Had Dior not been beyond my budget at the time, I would likely have become a customer. Like chic French women, I choose the best quality I can *afford*.

Chic French women may be using more natural and organic skin care, but they have not tossed out their Lancôme, Clinique, Nuxe, Dior, Guerlain, Avéne, Clarins and certainly not their Sisley. Who would throw out a tiny 1.7 oz. vial of anti-aging night treatment that cost $750? Toss that night treatment and a jar of Sisley's Global Anti-Age Cream at $460, and you have effectively bid adieu to more than $1200. Besides, who could toss products of a company, when the general manager who sets new standards for French male handsomeness tells *The New York Times* with great sincerity, "We try to provide answers to problems of everyday life, to make the customer more comfortable with herself, with the aging process."

Today many chic French women use a mix of products. Their natural and organic skin care products with their EcoCert and CosméBio certification logos along with commercial products with their chemical ingredients. Of course, the "classic" French cosmetic brands have long been high in botanicals. The difference in the ingredients in a natural or organic product might not be very different from a "classic" cosmetic product.

Nourishing plant oils are popular, certainly argan oil, one or the world's rarest oils that grows almost exclusively in Morocco. But almond oil is the plant oil in the very popular Nuxe *Huile Prodigieuse*, a dry oil spray that can be used on the face, body and hair. Not only does is this spray convenient and works well, but apparently it smells delicious.

Chic French women also like convenience. In the popular hyaluronic creams and serums that do a nice job (at least for a few hours) of disguising wrinkles, those in a roll-on are highly popular. Since many French women do not wear lipstick, lip balms are a must-have item, especially for certain age lips that often need plumping and smoothing. Lipsticks and lip balms (*baumes*) that contain hyaluronic acids can give nice pouty lips.

Skin care for chic women in France and the USA has much in common in techniques and products. When it comes to makeup, French and American women often see things quite differently.

A Note From Anne Barone

ABOUT BRANDS MENTIONED

In this book, in order to provide you with more specific and useful information, I have mentioned a number of specific companies, brands, services and products.

Please understand that mentioning specific companies, products, services, organizations or authorities in this book does not imply my endorsement. Nor does mention of specific companies, products, services, organizations or authorities imply that they endorse this book, its author, or its publisher.

With many of these products and services I mention, I have no personal experience. In the instances when I have used a particular product or service, I state that usage. Additionally, during the writing of this book, I have been trying a number of the products mentioned—to the noticeable improvement in my problem skin, I am happy to write. On the *Chic & Slim* website I will be sharing with readers some of my experiences with these (many French) products I have tried. Visit *annebarone.com* for more information.

Makeup

JUST AS CHIC FRENCH WOMEN want more naturalness from esthetic interventions to the aging process than most American women, they also want a more natural look in their makeup. Not true that chic French women do not wear makeup. French women just do not wear makeup that makes them look as if they are wearing makeup.

Chic French women do not want their beauty efforts and the money they spend on beauty products and treatments to be obvious. They want their beauty to appear "natural."

To chic French women "painted" faces look cheap, sending out a strong sexual message like a hooker. In their system, a woman does not use makeup to cover up skin problems, she uses good skin care to prevent or eliminate skin problems so that she has a tight-pored, luminous skin that needs no camouflage. The face reflecting the woman within. For the French, an overly made-up look gives a woman the appearance of *une poupée*, a babydoll. Luminous, meaning not only glowing, but also intellectual brilliance and enlightened, says here is a knowledgeable woman of substance and opinions. As Elaine Sciolino wrote in *"Sans Makeup, S'il Vous Plaît"* in *The New York Times*:

> On the whole, French women like to portray themselves

as more balanced, more inclined to pamper themselves and take pleasure in daily rituals than Americans. In its most extreme, America is seen as a youth-obsessed, throwaway, quick-fix culture where women are more likely to look artificially young and totally "done."

So at all ages, chic French women usually will not wear foundation makeup, *fond de teint*. They will especially avoid it in certain age because they think foundation makeup would make them look older by making lines and wrinkles more noticeable. Not surprising that when French women do wear something like a foundation, it might be one of the barely detectable mineral makeups or a gel or powder bronzer. They may let the sunscreen built into the bronzer or their day face treatment suffice for sun protection.

Chic French women and their dermatologists are not as determined as American women and their dermatologists that every ray of sunshine must be, at all cost, prevented from touching their skin, particularly their faces. One factor in this greater sun tolerance is that the closer to the equator you live, the stronger the sun's rays. Most people in the USA, especially those of us who live in the Sun Belt, require more skin protection than is necessary in France.

The French also recognize that the human body has bodily processes for good health, such as the making of Vitamin D for healthy bones, that are enhanced by sun exposure. Certainly sun abuse should be avoided. But with caution, some sun exposure can be tolerated. As for the wrinkles that sun exposure can cause, many chic French women are comfortable with them as the faces of any number of well-known French actresses of certain age testify.

Not that chic French women ignore the problems too much

sun can cause. At the time I was learning chic French women's approach to eating well and staying slim, I was also learning their techniques for moderation in sun exposure in those pre-sun protection product days. As the days warmed, gradual exposure to prevent burning was the rule. Especially near water, sun exposure before 10 AM and not until after 4 PM was another rule. Other times of day one stayed under a cabana or beach umbrella and always under a big hat. Remember that iconic photo of Pablo Picasso carrying the big beach umbrella over the head of the beautiful young woman in ankle length dress and big straw hat on the Riviera beach? That photo beautifully illustrates the classic French approach to sun exposure. By the way, that young woman in the hat shaded by Picasso's umbrella is the chic French artist Françoise Gilot, now 89, whom I wrote about in an earlier section of this book.

When asked by her *France Soir* interviewer what makeup she chose to harmonize with her naturally gray hair, novelist Tatiana de Rosnay said she never wore foundation, but she did use a little *Terracotta de Guerlain*, a bronzing powder, over Avène anti-redness cream. With this, a little Bourjois blush, a touch of mascara and Dior Ultra Gloss 212. The Avène cream has a SPF25, but the bronzing powder is without sunscreen. Even with what Tatiana de Rosnay describes as her "English skin," she apparently finds SPF 25 sufficient for going about her day.

The actress and Nice city councilwoman Sophie Duez told her interviewer that she usually did not wear foundation makeup, but when she did she liked YSL Perfect Touch. She finds the built-in applicator handy. Her sunscreen is Sisley's *le Grand Écran Solaire Visage* SPF 30 *ambré*. Sisley is the global company dedicated to quality cosmetics headed by the Hubert and Isabelle d'Ornano. When Daphne Merkin interviewed the d'Ornanos in July for *The New York Times* at their Quai D'Orsay apartment overlooking the

Seine, the writer noted that the Polish-born Isabelle d'Ornano's skin was lightly bronzed, and commented: "She is not as virulently anti-sun as most skin-care professionals, believing in moderate exposure with appropriate SPF protection."

The elegant Isabelle d'Ornano who regularly makes the international Best Dressed lists apparently does not aspire to the Sisterhood of the Marble Goddess Faces. But she does care for her skin with her company's carefully researched products. Daphne Merkin comments on her "aesthetic sensibility in which glowing skin is a part of the well-considered life rather than an arena of female obsession and anxiety." Hubert and Isabelle d'Ornano's son Philippe, Sisley's general manager, says that American women are focused on wrinkles rather than on the radiance of their skin.

Radiance is the more important to chic French women who worry less about wrinkles and also feel comfortable with faces without foundation makeup. The interviewer for the *Independent* noted about actress Juliette Binoche, 47, that her certain age face was "truly luminescent despite being scrubbed clean of make-up."

Part of the classic, natural French look for all ages is no, or hardly any noticeable eyeliner, but strong, dark, well-groomed eyebrows. Thinning eyebrows are one of those signs of certain age that should not be neglected. Yet, unless the correction is done with a degree of subtlety, it can look unnatural. You can solve the problem economically with brow powders and pencils, or you can go the more expensive permanent cosmetics route.

For that natural look, choosing the correct brush and brow powder shade is essential. You may have to experiment before you find the brow powder shade and applicator that works best for you. If you have gray hairs mixed in with your darker eyebrow hairs, you can tweeze these out if there are just one or two and they are determined to grow at bizarre angles. You can also buy eyebrow tints on wands that are safe to use near your eyes. While it is not safe to use hair color to dye eyebrows or lashes, there are safe products specifically designed for such use. Eyelash and brow tinting is probably a job you want done by an experienced professional at a salon, however.

A slanted bristled eyebrow brush is often recommended, but I get a more satisfactory result with one of those brow groomer brushes that have brush bristles on one side and a little comb on the other. I use that brush for applying brow powder for street makeup and use a brow pencil for more defined brows for photos. Though if needed, I help the powder out with a bit of pencil even for everyday makeup.

Permanent cosmetics tattoo on a pretty eyebrow. The work here in the USA I have seen looks natural and is a great time saver for busy women whose every minute of the day must be carefully budgeted. Permanent cosmetics are certainly offered at French beauty institutes.

Mascara is a must for chic French women. Each has their favorite brand. For removing mascara and other eye makeup, a bestseller, at least for mass distribution, is Gemey-Maybelline *Cils Demasq.* Gemey-Maybelline is the French incarnation of Maybelline we know so well in the USA. And *cils demasq* is that Maybelline eye makeup remover we also know well.

As I mentioned in the previous section, chic French women favor more subtle lip balm and gloss over lipstick. A problem in certain age is that the lips get thinner. Even if you don't want to go the injection route with expensive fillers, there are any number of inexpensive lip plumper products combined with a touch of color that can give certain age lips a more youthful look. If you want to spend the money, you can also have permanent color applied to your lips.

At the time that permanent cosmetics became popular, three friends banded together for moral support and all went the same day to the same technician to have eyebrows, eyeliner and lip color. I saw the photos taken shortly after my friends' work. If I had not known all three husbands for decades, I would have taken one look at those immediately-after photos and thought them abused wives. Of course, the swelling was temporary. The three husbands, by the way, expressed approval of the permanent cosmetics. They liked having their wives with prettily made up eyes and rosy lips 24/7. They approved so much that they didn't even complain about the hundreds of dollars the permanent makeup cost. You would almost think those husbands were French.

IN THE FUTURE, there will be only one face. And if the Oscars are predictive, there will be only one body—big chest, skinny body— and one style. In decades past, each top glamour girl aimed for a signature face and measurements, a trademark voice, a unique walk. You never saw Katharine Hepburn and Ava Gardner showing up in the same dress, or Audrey Hepburn and Marilyn Monroe looking like a pair of matching candles.

As Shakespeare wrote of the ultimate glamour girl, Cleopatra: "Age cannot wither her, nor custom stale her infinite variety."

Women have become so fixated on not withering, they've forgotten that there are infinite ways to be beautiful.

Maureen Dowd
Frozen Mermaids, Scary Sirens
in *The New York Times*

Teeth

DURING THE LAST FRENCH PRESIDENTIAL CAMPAIGN, the Socialist candidate, chic Ségolène Royal, 57, had a tooth straightened. Howls of criticism arose from the public and the media. The French have never gone in for cosmetic dentistry the way Americans have. Anyone whose face appears in the American media is expected to have perfectly straight, gleaming white teeth. But the French feel the same way about that level of cosmetic dentistry as they do about American women who have extensive facial work done to give them Marble Goddess Faces. Actually, the candidate's sin according to the way the French think was not that Ségolène Royal had her tooth straightened, but that she did it at a time when it was noticed.

One change in chic French women over the past several decades is that they are now smiling, big broad smiles. On television, in photos, in advertising, in political campaigns. Even Catherine Deneuve has given up the icy demeanor for which she was long known. You see her on television and she is laughing and smiling. When you smile widely, of course your teeth are on view. I always thought the reason French women did not smile much was their teeth. These women wore impeccable clothes with chic hair and accessories, but there was sometimes a crooked tooth or two. Smoking and that dark strong French coffee stained teeth. These days French women are smiling, and the teeth we see are usually white and straight. The odds are there has been some dental help. But done when no one noticed.

Certain age often brings an increase in dental problems. The good news is that today's dentistry is able with implants and other techniques to restore most mouths from whatever accidents, incompetent dentistry and other disasters that may have befallen it over the years. The bad news is that this dental work is *very* expensive and that unless you are selective, you may have some very expensive work done poorly. I can tell you from sad experience there are a LOT of incompetent dentists.

You may have a regular dentist you love, but he will likely refer you to specialists for complicated extractions, crowns, bridges, implants and such. Be cautious that his referral is not just a woman who was in his class in dental school or the guy he plays golf with on Friday. Make sure this is a dentist who will do more good than harm to your mouth. Do your research. Wikipedia and professional dental organization websites have good information about oral surgery, implants, and other dental services. Know what you are getting into. Know the total cost. In the consultations for dental work I have been having lately, I have found that when you start discussing price, they give you a figure for the basic service, extraction, bridge or whatever. But some dentists do not include in this figure anesthesia and other related services. You may find your total bill substantially higher than your initial quote.

When you go to dentists today and they talk about your "teeth," that's cleaning, fillings, root canals and such. Plain old dentistry. When they start talking about your "smile," they want to sell you $55,000 worth of cosmetic dentistry.

Cosmetic dentistry has reached a point where by changing the angle of the teeth and other techniques. a cosmetic dentist can correct for some aging changes and give a more youthful face. If you are having major restorative work done anyway, check out these techniques. For the same price, or a fraction more than "functional," you might get "prettier" and "more youthful."

The seemingly unavoidable problem for certain age teeth is the darkening that comes as part of the aging process. Dentists have a variety of solutions, principal among them whitening procedures and veneers. There are also several economical products and techniques you can employ without professional services.

Years past dentists would tell their certain age patients to switch from their regular toothpaste to bicarbonate of soda (baking soda), or in half and half combination with table salt. Now we know brushing with these should only be done once a week because of the danger of damaging tooth enamel. Of course we have all those "whitening" toothpastes that work better for some than others. There are also toothpastes such as Sensodyne's Pronamel designed to protect the enamel of the teeth for those who eat or drink highly acidic foods and beverages.

If you drink a lot of coffee, or hot tea as I do, stains from these can be a problem. Just as can stains from healthy fruits such as blueberries or blackberries. A corrective for these stains I like is Paula's Choice brighten up 2-minute teeth whitener. It comes in a small tube like a lipstick and you paint it on the front of your visible teeth. No rinsing is needed. Works well on my tea-stained or berry-stained teeth and tastes good too.

A trick for making teeth appear whiter is to use a blue-toned lipstick to give the optical illusion of whiter teeth. Whatever you use, be aware that white teeth can give you a more youthful—and certainly more attractive—smile.

Eyes

FOR MY GENERATION OF AMERICAN FEMALES, lipstick and high heels proclaimed the transition from childhood to adolescence. Reading glasses suspended from a chain around the neck, or for the hipper among us reading glasses parked on the top our heads, proclaimed our transition into certain age. Men can ignore the reality of presbyopia, that certain age vision change, for more years than women. They have longer arms to hold the print further from their eyes.

For those who, in younger years, enjoyed perfect vision, this gradual change in vision can sneak up, especially on those who have an inclination for denial. I enjoyed extraordinarily good vision in my early adult years. But one doctor who examined me mid-20s had warned, "You have great vision now, but when you reach middle age, you will have to wear trifocals, and it will be almost impossible to get the prescription right."

Lucky for me that by the time I was ready for those trifocals the doctor who forecast vision doom had mentioned, multifocal contacts had been invented. By choosing carefully, I found a doctor who was able to prescribe correction that gave me vision as good as I had in my 20s. For me contact lenses are so comfortable that as long as I stay away from ceiling fans and out of high wind and blowing dust, I am usually unaware I am wearing corrective lenses. Yet between my era of perfect vision and my multifocal contact lenses, there was a progression through reading glasses and even a time with monovision contact lenses. That is wearing one contact for seeing up close and the other for distance vision.

As I suggested a few paragraphs earlier, the onset and worsening of presbyopia and the need for correction comes on gradually. In my early 40s I began to notice that long sessions at the computer made my eyes tired and sometimes gave me headaches. I had a pair of reading glasses with some 1X magnification and these worked for a couple of years. Then, I decided it was time to spend the money on an eye exam and have prescription reading glasses made.

I found an eye doctor, had an exam. Three days after I got my new reading glasses, the left ear piece came off in my hand. The hinge holding the ear piece onto the main part of the eyeglasses was missing the pin. I took the new reading glasses back to the optician who had made them. I expected the repair to take a few minutes, but the technician said it would take several days. When I went to pick up my eyeglasses, a smiling technician said, "We got those lenses changed out for you."

"Lenses? It was the ear piece that was the problem."

"No, no, no," he insisted. The problem was the lenses weren't ground to the correct prescription. I looked at the glasses. The right lens was twice as thick as the left and too thick to fit completely inside the frame surrounding it. The eyeglasses looked hideous.

"But those two lenses are different thicknesses," I said.

The technician looked sheepish. "I know. But your eyes are different."

Not that different.

Not only did the glasses look hideous, I could not see well through the new lenses. The ear piece still wouldn't stay on.

The next week I was still bickering with the optician over the glasses when I went to lunch with some women I knew. At the table two of the women were discussing how each had prescription reading glasses made and they could not see to read with them so they had gone to Dillard's and bought Liz Claiborne readers.

I decided my battle with the optician probably was not worth more of my time and effort. I went to Dillard's and bought Liz Claiborne readers. With them I could see to read and work at the computer. The frames were sturdy and fit perfectly. Unable to get my money back from the optician, I donated the glasses to an organization where volunteer technicians regrind old glasses to the prescription of people too poor to buy eyeglasses. I hope they had some tape for that ear piece.

In a couple of years, my presbyopia worsened beyond only wearing glasses for reading and work at the computer. If that doctor in my 20s was right and it would be tricky getting the prescription right, I decided I had better stick with my reading glasses rather than try my luck with another eye doctor and optician. I had some 2.5X readers for work at the computer and reading and 1X for driving and walking around. Inconvenient switching between them, but I could see, and I was not wasting hundreds of dollars on badly-made eyeglasses.

If you don't want to wear reading glasses, you have some options once presbyopia sets in. President Reagan popularized the wearing of one contact lens. A friend who tried the system as soon as she learned of it, praised it highly. If your vision is still adequate for distance, you can wear one contact lens for viewing up close. The one contact lens à la Reagan is a more modern version of the monocle popular in the early 20th century.

Another early 20th century option for presbyopia correction was the lorgnette. When two lenses were needed, but the elegant woman did not wish to wear eyeglasses, only have them at hand when needed, her choice was these eyeglasses on a stick. The lorgnette folded together like a jackknife when not in use. If you have seen certain movies of the 1930s and 1940s, there is sometimes a grande dame that whips out her lorgnette and peers imperiously.

If you were really into vintage fashion, when you reach certain age, you might scour antique and collectible shops for a monocle or lorgnette with suitable magnification. I have a pair of elegant gold wire frame bifocals inherited from a great aunt. Genetics being what they are, the prescription is so exactly mine at this age that I can wear them. They are rimless with elegant gold nose bridge and ear pieces. The bifocal lens instead of covering almost the lower half are small and centered, like an elegant little beveled pane in the center of each lens.

Bifocals with the visible line do say age. But for more money you now have progressive lens that are indistinguishable from regular glasses that younger people wear. With the choice of attractive frames, eyeglasses can be sexy and fashionable. The selection of chic, stylish frames is extensive.

From my own experience, even with a good prescription of progressive lenses, I don't have as accurate correction as I do with my multifocal contacts lenses. Especially if it is necessary to look down over uneven footing. With progressive bifocals, a computer screen needs careful placement so you don't have to tilt your head backward to be able to see though the lower section of the eyeglass lens. Many people who must work long hours at the computer, when they reach certain age, opt for specially prescribed computer glasses that they wear only for computer work. Instead you might buy a computer stand that places your computer at the right height for your eyes. You would probably find it considerably less expensive to buy a stand for your computer than to buy a special pair of prescription lenses for computer work.

There is now a corrective surgery for some presbyopia, I understand. But I have never known anyone who had the surgery, nor even read articles advocating it as a better solution than eyeglasses or contact lenses.

Chic French women of certain age seem to opt more often for contact lenses than eyeglasses. Or else they whip off their bifocals whenever in camera range. Two who make stylish eyeglasses a fashion accessory are former government minister Michèle Alliot-Marie and writer Michèle Fitoussi.

DRY EYES ARE ANOTHER PROBLEM that often comes with certain age. That burning, feels-as-if-there-is-sand-in-the-eye sensation is a greater problem for women than men. Menopausal changes, as well as lengthy sessions at the computer screen, and certain prescription medications can be causative factors.

In many cases, over-the-counter artificial tears along with frequent glancing away from the computer screen, wearing sunglasses, blinking and eating more foods with beneficial omega-3s and omega-6s such as flaxseed oil will take care of the symptoms, according to Mary Duenwald who wrote on the subject in *The New York Times*.

Like other eye problems that come as part of certain age, dry eyes have a number of remedies. You just have to find the ones that work best for your eye health and comfort. And chic. Don't neglect chic.

Ears

PREVIOUSLY, THE SAME REASON for the prohibition against long hair on women of certain age applied to large hoop and long dangling earrings on women of certain age. These accessories were thought to "pull the face down" as well as call attention to sagging skin on the neck and thus make signs of aging more apparent. But today you see chic French women of certain age wearing hoop earrings of full dimensions and ornate concoctions of stones and metal that dangle to the shoulder. They look great—though a tad exotic. How successfully an older woman can wear longer ear ornamentation depends on her face, her hair, the totality of her personal style—and her earlobes.

By the time some women pass the 50-year mark, those neat little holes in the earlobe made lo those decades ago when you first had your ears pierced are now long vertical slits that are testimony to the years. A cosmetic dermatologist can return these slits to neat little holes.

But if you are not inclined to pay $600 and go six weeks without your earrings while healing, you can sometimes put a tiny bit of surgical tape behind your ear and then poke the post of a light-weight earring through the surgical tape. The tape will keep the post from sliding down to the bottom of the slit. I have at times been more successful at making this work than others. In any case, at best it is a short term fix.

From a personal style viewpoint, ears are a point of accessorizing. Their more important function, of course, are the mechanism inside the ear for hearing. As far as I can learn, there is little one can do to prevent the changes in the eye that happen with age. But if you take some basic precautions earlier in your life, hearing loss in one's later years is not absolute, specialists in audiology now tell us. Prevention of loss requires consistently protecting your ears from loud noise.

I finally realized I was being so conscientious wearing earplugs when I mowed the lawn or used other loud outdoor equipment. But I was surely exposing my hearing to more possible damage from my extremely noisy blender and vacuum cleaner.

A variety of earplugs are available, and I have tried several different designs. The ones that worked best for me were earplugs on a cord that fits around the neck so you don't drop them if you have to take them out. They can be cleaned easily and disinfected for future use and stored in a little container. Inexpensive so you can have several pair in locations you might need them.

If despite precautions you still end up with hearing loss, technology in hearing aids is getting better. Though no one I know who uses them has ever claimed that these devices gave hearing equal to that before their loss. The good aids are costly.

In any case, constantly asking people to repeat what they say, or constantly saying "eh?" is not chic. But you can take comfort that a great deal of what people say is not important. You may not be missing much in what you do not hear. If you have noisy neighbors, you might even consider hearing loss a blessing.

Neck

WHEN WRITER NORA EPHRON REACHED CERTAIN AGE, she felt extremely distressed about her neck with its signs of age worsened by the clumsy work from a previous surgery for possible cancer. Instead of cosmetic surgery, the screenwriter who gave us *Sleepless in Seattle* and *You've Got Mail*, wrote an essay about her neck and made it the lead in her book *I Feel Bad About My Neck*. Nora Ephron still feels bad about her neck, but at least she enjoyed the earnings and success of a bestseller.

Olivia Goldsmith, author of *The First Wives Club*, and veteran of other cosmetic surgeries was also distressed about her certain age neck. She did choose surgery. The *Times* (UK) wrote about the writer's death during "a wholly unnecessary procedure to smooth the skin on her neck."

During surgery to remove a flap of skin from her neck at Manhattan's Lenox Hill hospital, the 54-year-old novelist suffered a heart attack and lapsed into a coma. Late last week she died, never having regained consciousness. So instead of celebrating her enhanced looks with a fashionable décolleté dress or a dazzling row of diamonds, Goldsmith lies on a mortuary slab.

Harshly worded. But the point is made that despite the relative safety of cosmetic surgery today, there are risks. Some are even life and death risks.

Beyond their skin care routines and treatments at the *instituts de beauté*, the solution to aging necks for chic French women of certain age have long been those traditional French fashion icons: turtlenecks and scarves. Like American women, French women also use choker necklaces and little jackets with mandarin collars. Chic French women have an interesting riff on the mandarin collar technique. They wear the jackets open down to their bra, or where their bra or camisole would be if they wore one, which often they don't. That bared décolletage is another example of using a tantalizing distraction to lead eyes away from a feature they don't want noticed. And of course that décolletage has been creamed and peeled into skin as luminous as their faces.

As far as I can learn, no chic French woman of certain age has written a book about feeling bad about her neck. They are too busy writing books with titles such as *Without Regrets* (Bourdin), *The Woman Who Invented The Beauty Business* (Fitoussi) *Who Were You Thinking Of When You Were Making Love To Me?* (Chapsal).

As far as I can learn, no chic French woman has died in any event relating directly to her certain age neck. At least not since France retired the guillotine.

MORE INFORMATION
About Living *Chic & Slim*
Chic & Slim Website

annebarone.com

Arms

IN A RECENT REVIEW of French actress Isabelle Huppert's new film *White Material*, reviewer for *The New York Times*, Manohla Dargis describes a scene where the actress is hanging off the back of a bus. "As she holds on tight, her short-sleeved dress fluttering, the camera moves in close enough for you to see the muscles in Ms. Huppert's thin arms popping, straining with the terrific effort that encapsulates the will to survive." No flabby upper arms for this chic French woman aged 57.

How does Isabelle Huppert avoid that scourge of certain age, loose skin on upper arms? Who knows? Though the actress has never been hesitant to bare her body to the public, she generally keeps personal information under wraps.

Not true that French women do not exercise. They can be regular in their toning routines, for instance a short workout with hand weights for upper arms. And then, of course, there are all those treatments at the *instituts de beauté* and spas to help the process along.

Alberta-born Nancy Huston, also 57, who is chic—and French by long permanent residence—is forthcoming about how she keeps her upper arms in shape. During an interview session with the *Independent's* Gerry Feehily, with the Metro car's door shutting before they could enter, the writer grasped the doors with her hands and wrenched them back open, explaining: "I do weights."

Keeping certain age upper arms toned takes only a few minutes a day. But you must be regular about the exercise. I use hand weights. Sometime around age 50 my mother acquired a rope contraption that hooked to her bedroom door with which she religiously did a short, daily workout session. Looking at a photo of her lifting her toddler grandson you can see the well-toned muscles of her 57-year old arms. The contraption worked.

Whatever equipment or routine you choose, you must do it regularly to have those shapely upper arms.

If you don't want to bother with exercise, you can wear sleeves that come to the elbow. If you can't buy this sleeve length in the style and color you like, it is easy to cut off and hem long sleeves to the precise length you want. British actress Helen Mirren does the best job of finding formal dresses that cleverly cover certain age arms. Look at photos of Helen Mirren at awards ceremonies and you will see some clever fashion solutions to the problem.

In certain age, not only the skin and muscles of the arms require attention. Problems can arise in underarms as well. In my late 40s, my underarm deodorant began to cause irritation. I changed brands—several times. Still irritation. I switched to a natural brand. No irritation, but unfortunately it was not effective when challenged by stress or Texas summer heat.

Finally in an article in *The New York Times* beauty section I found an herbal underarm deodorant developed for the Israeli Army that was aluminum-free and only needed to be applied about once a week. I ordered a jar. I have used Lavilin for several years now. It works. And the about once-a-week application is convenient.

Hands

IN DIANE JOHNSON'S NOVEL *Le Divorce*, an American woman in Paris who is writing a book on French women comments on the appearance of another American, the Californian Roxy, now married to a Frenchman and living in Paris. "She always looks so awful," says the writer. And what contributes to Roxy's awfulness, according to French women's standards against which the writer is measuring? Roxy wears jeans "like an American" and no scarf. But the greatest of her sins is that Roxy does not take proper care of her nails.

Chic French women believe well-maintained and well-manicured hands are very important.

For all ages of chic French women that means regular creaming to keep hands soft and smooth and regular attention to nails to keep them neat and well-shaped. The major French skin care companies make hand creams, Nuxe has a hand and nail cream with Chilean rose, avocado and sweet almond oil. There are dozens by the companies that make natural and organic products. Weleda has wild rose, iris, and pomegranate. L'Occitane en Provence offers hand creams in orange blossom, vanilla, winter rose, lavender, and cherry blossom. Laura Mercier, *Crème de Pistache*. And Clarins sells *Fluide Anti-Tache Jeunesse des Mains*,

Liquid Anti-Spots Youthfulness of Hands with SPF 15. For certain age hands, if the hand cream does not contain sunscreen—and most don't—rubbing sunscreen on the backs of your hands may be necessary to protect against age spots. Gardening gloves are a must. Atlas makes reasonably-priced gardening gloves that fit like a second skin and give you dexterity for your outdoor chores.

A hand cream that you may find tucked in the hand bag of chic French women is not a hand cream *per se*. It is Boiron Calendula Cream, an homeopathic product made by the French company Boiron that has wide distribution in the USA. You can find the calendula cream at Target, or likely your drugstore. The cream soothes chapped hands and can be emergency treatment for minor burns and cuts.

Chic French women, especially those of certain age, will be likely to have shiny buffed nails, not polished. If they do wear nail polish, it will likely be clear or pearly rather than colored. Part of the reason for avoiding colored nail polish is chic French women's tendency toward the simple and natural that we have discussed earlier in this book. Maintenance between manicures is easier with buffed nails or those with clear polish. Another reason is the belief that wearing nail polish, except for special very dressed-upped times, is damaging to the nails.

Bastien Gonzalez is currently the reining nail expert in Paris. He advises his clients to avoid wearing nail polish on a regular basis because polish can dry out and damage the nails as can the polish remover that will be required to remove the polish. Additionally color pigments in nail polish can burn the nails and make them yellow. He advises using a glass nail file (you can wash it for better hygiene) and buffing nails after applying a nail buffing cream.

Beyond age spots, certain age hands can become wrinkled, bony, and the veins prominent. Restylane and Juvéderm fillers can give short term correction. But many who are truly disturbed about signs of age of their hands opt for fat transfer in which a cosmetic surgeon harvests fat from an area of a person's body where there is an excess of fat and inserts it into the hands. That takes care of wrinkled and bony.

For the noticeable blue veins that signal "old lady hands," there are a couple of procedures. First there is sclerotherapy in which the veins are injected with a drug that burns the inner lining of the vein causing it to clot off and eventually scar down. This same technique is used for leg veins. Unfortunately, sometimes sclerotherapy can leave an unwanted brown stain.

Another technique is avulsions of hand veins in which veins are removed from the hands. The three women who described their experience with this procedure for the *Daily Mail* (UK) were pleased with their new younger-looking hands. The experience under local anesthesia in which an incision was made in the hand and the veins pulled out with a little hook was not much fun for any of them. And one of the three was not sure she would go back for the second hand. Even with anesthesia, the women said they could feel the veins being pulled.

In the USA, it is apparently possible to have the procedure done less painfully. According to his website, Dr. Lawrence P. Mueller who does a similar hand avulsion procedure in his Merced, California clinic takes a two-step approach to minimize pain and risk. Only one or two disfiguring hand veins are removed at a time. Half the veins are removed first, then, six to eight weeks later, the remaining veins are removed. Advantages of the two-stage approach allows the deeper veins time to adjust to the increased blood flow now diverted to them. It also reduces the risk of hand swelling and dilation of other veins. Swelling and discoloration are usually gone in one or two weeks.

My own prize for the most inventive solution to the problem of aging hands goes to fashion designer Karl Lagerfeld. He is never photographed without his fingerless gloves of which he seems to have an endless assortment made in different colors and materials. Whatever signs of aging there may be on his hands, they are covered by the gloves. (And whatever signs of aging around his eyes are covered by those dark glasses he always wears.) Those gloves also keep his hands warm. Mr. Lagerfeld's solution is a reminder that in the days when ladies wore little white gloves, besides providing a formality and elegance to their appearance, those gloves covered age spots on hands.

HER LOOK IS DAZZLINGLY SIMPLE and make-up and accessories are hardly to be seen. In the space of just two consummately handled public appearances, she has simultaneously managed to restore the international reputation of French chic and modernise it—while also standing as a shining example of how not to make being Almost-Fifty matter one jot. No accident, one is sure—though the coup de grace is that she made it look as if she wasn't trying too hard. That, of course, is the elusive essence of "understated" French insouciance—the thing that, as she proved, in contrast with her pretty girls, only gets better in amazing Parisian middle-age.

Sarah Mower *writing about Cecilia Sarkozy*
Cecilia, you're breaking our hearts
in *Telegraph.co.uk*

Legs

HOW DO THOSE CHIC FRENCH WOMEN OF CERTAIN AGE have those *ooh-la-la* legs?

Most chic French women stay slim. That takes care the basic problem. But even slim thighs can suffer that dimpling the French have long called cellulite or that *peau d'orange*, orange peel skin. Legs of any size and toning can suffer unsightly broken veins. How do chic French women keep cellulite and broken veins from disfiguring their legs?

The first of three basic elements in chic French leg care is a good daily program. As with facial care, chic French women begin early, even in their teens. They often use products specifically created to prevent and treat leg problems.

Second, if they can possibly afford it, chic French women get professional help keeping their legs in good health and appearance and with treating any problems that occur. *Instituts des jambes*, leg institutes, specialize in leg treatments. Specialist physicians and estheticians using traditional manual, as well as high tech equipment, treat cellulite and circulatory problems, underlying causes of broken veins. Estheticians at regular *instituts de beauté* also give specialized treatments for legs.

The third factor in beautiful French legs is that, as soon as any sign of leg problems arise, chic French women take action. They never assume that if they just ignore it, the problem will clear up on its own.

What regular leg maintenance do chic French women do?

Interestingly, diet and lifestyle recommendations to promote healthy blood circulation of the legs are much the same as those the French advise to prevent cellulite. Avoid excessive sugar, salt, alcohol and tobacco. Eat lots of fresh fruits and vegetables for vitamin C and antioxidants, plant oils for vitamin E. Drink plenty of water, six to eight glasses a day. Avoid tight clothing. Keeping their legs pretty is a reason why many French women do not wear underpants or panty hose that would restrict circulation. If they do wear tight jeans or other restrictive clothing, when at home they wear something loose-fitting such a slip or robe to compensate.

Of course chic French women do all that healthy walking, the best exercise for legs. Whenever you see a chic French woman sitting in a sidewalk cafe, remind yourself that she probably arrived there via a brisk walk and will make the return to home or to work on her feet, the way she came. As articles in the American media do, French publications remind women if sitting for long periods, at a desk or for plane or train travel for instance, that at least every hour they should do several minutes of stretching exercises such as ankle rotations to keep the blood circulating well.

Certain herbal remedies are thought to help in the battle against cellulite and vein problems. Bilberry, butcher's broom, sweet clover and blackcurrant are available in infusions (teas) or capsules.

Another element in the daily care program that I must confess I have neglected are the cold showers and baths. Chic French women believe that hot water causes circulatory problems and thus broken veins in the legs. Just as they treat their breasts to a daily spray of cold (not icy) water for toning, they also give their legs a toning spraying once at day—or, as some leg specialists advise—twice a day. According to information in a special feature *de belle jambes*, beautiful legs on the website *auFeminin.com*, this procedure assumes that the shower has one of those shower heads attached to a hose that can be handheld. Holding the spray of cold water about four inches from the skin, the spray should begin at the big toe and progresses upward to the inside of the knee, then descend on the outside of the leg down to the ankle. To treat the legs in a bathtub, the instructions are to extend the leg and spray with cool (thank goodness, not cold) water from the ankle to the hip. This is to be continued alternating legs until the water in the tub is up to the thighs—or if you can stand it, the waist. These cold showers and baths are not too unpleasant in hot weather. Perhaps they are unnecessary in cold weather when the outside temperatures provide a cold air bath every time one ventures outdoors.

Commercial leg sprays can be purchased, or you can distill your own from herbal recipes. These sprays can be carried in the purse and used on the legs when the circulation might need a boost. (Here's another reason chic French women choose to be bare-legged.) A popular leg spray is Dr. Hauschka's Rosemary Leg & Arm Toner that promises to reduce the appearance of varicose veins and cellulite and also stimulate the skin. At about a third the price of Dr. Hauschka's leg spray is Foot & Leg Spa Mist by the American company Aromafloria. This spray is designed to cool, deodorize, and work against inflammation.

Daily leg massages are also important to keep legs pretty. These massages are usually done immediately after bathing with products designed to tone the skin and improve circulation. These massages should always begin at the extremity and work toward the heart, in this case, at the ankle and working up to the top of the thigh. Some find applying a leg cream after a dry brushing improves circulation.

If a separate foot balm is used, then the foot would be massaged first. But many products are designed to be used for both foot and leg. If using one of those or just a general skin lotion, the massage would begin with the foot not ankle. Botanicals are active ingredients in these products. While many chic French women would use their preferred body lotion or massage oil, many products specially designed for leg massage are also popular. On the higher end are Clarins *Anti-Eau* Body Treatment Oil that is designed to help "eliminate toxins and stimulate and firm skin." With essential oils of broom, geranium and marjoram, it claims to be especially beneficial to problem legs. *Tonific Minceur Gel-Crème* by Nuxe is targeted to the thigh portion of the leg for action against cellulite, flabby or "orange peel" skin. Popular and much more economical is Cattier's *Lotion Rafraîchissante*, Refleshing Lotion for Legs. This lotion is to be sprayed on clean dry skin in the evening and massaged in from ankle to thigh. Principal ingredients are peppermint and menthol. Even more budget-priced is Burt's Bees Peppermint Foot Lotion that also contains peppermint and menthol as principal ingredients.

For chic French women who wear those chic French high heels, this leg daily care routine is especially important. Pressure wearing those shoes puts on the ball of the foot impedes circulation in the legs. Chic French women may also pay astronomical sums for their stiletto heels because, beyond fashion, some of the name brands have a "comfort cushion" that helps to alleviate the pressure on the foot and thus not so likely to cause leg problems. For those who buy more economically priced high heels, toe pad inserts can be purchased at drug or discount store.

In the late 1970s, writer Linda Dannenberg spent a month in Paris having beauty treatments at the various salons and *instituts de beauté.* Many changes have occurred on the French beauty scene since her book based on her experience *The Paris Way of Beauty* was published in 1979. But two leg treatments she underwent at the Paris *Institut des Jambes* are still being used. Though the medically approved Frigibas does not sound like any more fun today than it was when Linda Dannenberg had those chilling wet stockings impregnated with a special hypothermatic liquid pulled on her legs 30 years ago. *La pressothérapie* sounds less uncomfortable. To-the-thigh inflatable booties apply an undulating pressure to the legs in a 30-minute treatment designed to stimulate circulation.

More recently on the anti-cellulite scene are various endermologie treatments in which an esthetician using a handheld device applies rolling, suction and massage to the skin. The idea is to increase circulation and break down unwanted fat cell deposits. The Cellu M6 program is an endermologie treatment popular in France (and the USA) and available at numerous *institut de beauté.*

The *Journal des Femmes* on *linternaute.com* gave a detailed account of a young French woman who underwent treatment with Cellu M6. This account provided insights into how chic French women seek professional treatment at the first sign of problems. At age 30, measuring 5 ft 5.5 inches (1,68 m) and 130 pounds (59 kg) the young woman was bothered by cellulite that had appeared on her thighs. In 20 sessions of 35 minutes, two per week for 10 weeks at her neighborhood *institut de beauté* she was treated for this problem. Encouraged by her progress after a few sessions with the Cellu M6, she decided to lower her caloric intake to subtract a few pounds during the treatment. She ate a breakfast of three slices of *pain aux céréales,* a whole grain bread currently popular in Paris, with yogurt and sliced fruit. Lunch was either sashimi, a combination salad, or roast chicken and vegetables. Supper was steamed green vegetables, two slices of *pain aux céréales,* and yogurt. She ate an apple as a snack later in the evening. She increased her exercise from 30 minutes per week to three sessions of 30 minutes. She also massaged in an anti-cellulite product daily. At the end of her treatment, each of her thighs saw a reduction of 3/4 inch (2 cm) in circumference. She thought her $680 (she caught a special that was 20 percent off the regular price) was well-spent and decided to go back for monthly maintenance treatments.

Of course, what went through my mind as I read this account (and likely is going through your mind as well) is whether this French woman would have achieved the same results with the endermologie treatment if she had kept her food intake and exercise the same as normal and not used the anti-cellulite product? Conversely, would she have had the same reduction in thigh measurement if she had only lowered her calorie intake, increased her exercise and used the anti-cellulite product? Chic French women do not ponder such questions. When they notice a problem, they bring on as much of the arsenal of remedies as their budgets will allow. Chic French women leave treatment evaluations to the research organizations. They concentrate on staying chic, slim and beautiful.

IN ADDITION TO THE HIGH TECH LEG TREATMENTS, numerous manual treatments specifically designed for legs and hips are also available. For example, at the Mosaic Spa at the Hilton, the Decléor Perfect Legs treatment begins with an exfoliation of the entire leg, then a massage with essential oils to aid circulation, a wrap with camphor and menthol, then *veinotoniques,* tonic of a circulation-aiding product, reflexology and then the application of a cooling gel.

Also, when it comes to leg beauty, chic French women never fail to take immediate action when they experience the slightest twinge of *jambes lourdes*. What exactly is *jambes lourdes*, heavy legs? Why do chic French women believe *jambes lourdes* is such a threat to beautiful legs?

Not so much a condition, as a sensation that an estimated 70 percent of French women suffer, especially during hot weather. French women describe this sensation as the feeling that each leg weighs a ton. Discomfort usually accompanies the feeling that the legs have suddenly morphed from flesh and bone into solid lead. Having experienced an unfortunate episode of *jambes lourdes* last summer, I believe the description of legs weighing a ton is accurate. *Jambes lourdes* is a warning signal of vein problems and those unsightly broken veins on the legs.

As for my own experience last August, the temperature was in the high 90s and pushing for a mid-day heat of 100+ degrees F. I had been mowing the lawn for three hours, staying well hydrated and taking a 15-minute break with legs elevated on an ottoman after the first hour and a half session. Coming into the house at the end of the three hours of mowing, I had the sensation that my legs weighed about a thousand pounds. Worse, there were stings on my thighs as if the veins were popping. I went immediately to the shower to cool down. Then I quickly got out my slant board and despite being hungry and really wanting lunch, I spent 30 minutes with my feet elevated 12 inches above my head to relieve the pressure on the veins.

Had I employed the full French system, I would have added several elements to the treatment. Immediately after cooling them down with the cold water, I would have done a leg massage with one of the products (and there are many) designed for *jambes lourdes*. For instance, Melvita's *Gel Jambes Légéges*, Gel for Light Legs (sold in English-speaking countries as Relaxing Leg Gel) has principal ingredients of menthol and rosemary with a number of other herbal ingredients. Generally, when you look for a product to relive a bout of *jambes lourdes*, you look for menthol, lemon or camphor to cool, and witch hazel, butcher's broom, cypress or horse chestnut extracts for benefit of the veins.

Had I been in France when I suffered the episode of *jambes lourdes*, I would have sought out one of the spa treatments designed to deal with the problem. And, of course, I would have continued to follow a daily leg care program with the elements mentioned earlier in this section. Too, I would have tried to follow the venerable prescription for leg care: *Never stand if you can sit. Never sit with feet on the floor if you can sit with feet elevated. Try to elevate your feet above your head at least 15 minutes to a half hour a day.* A slant board is convenient for this elevation. But you can also lie on the floor with a thin cushion under your head and put your feet up on the sofa or chair cushion with your knees bent at the edge of the cushion.

BUT WHAT DOES A CHIC FRENCH WOMAN DO if heredity or hormonal changes are too much for her vein problem prevention effort? The two remedies are treatment with lasers and treatment with sclerotherapy in which medicine is injected into the veins to make them shrink. While I have never had sclerotherapy, several years ago I had laser treatment for spider veins on my legs that was successful. I was careful to follow up the procedure by keeping off my feet and legs elevated for about two weeks afterward to help the process along. The treatment was relatively painless and moderately expensive.

Yet another solution for those who do not choose either sclerotherapy or zapping the unsightly veins with lasers is a wardrobe that hides leg problems: pants and opaque stockings. Chic French women have also long used leg makeup. The problem I always had with leg makeups was that they rubbed off on chairs and car seats. These days the best leg makeup is self tanner. Most self tanners today dry quickly, won't rub off after dry, and will build up color with regular use for even better camouflage of leg imperfections. Two inexpensive ones that work reasonably well are Sublime Bronze, L'Oréal Paris and the Jergens Natural Glow. A more specialized and more expensive tanner specifically for legs is *Gloss Bronzeur Jambes, Ambre Solaire Garnier.*

Certain age legs certainly have more challenges that younger legs. It can be discouraging when leg problems related to aging begin. Sometimes leg problems can be brought on by medication. When I was living on the Gulf Coast in that condominium, another resident I saw frequently at the pool had noticeably great legs. Remember Stockard Channing's legs in those short shorts in the film *Grease*? This woman had legs that good and she was almost 60. Then I noticed that almost overnight her legs became fat and flabby. She hadn't otherwise gained weight. What happened? A few days after I noticed this change, I met her returning from exercise. She told me she had just been for a five-mile hike. Shiny new leg weights were attached to her ankles.

The woman's leg problem had been caused by a medication her doctor prescribed. Horrified by what had happened so suddenly to disfigure her legs, she sought an equally speedy remedy. Unfortunately, she injured her leg muscles with that long hike the first time out with leg weights.

When you set out to correct leg problems with exercise, do so gradually and with caution. Also, make sure that you carefully research any treatment you pursue to make sure that it is the right one for you.

Chic French women of certain age have great legs, and you can have great legs too following their system.

Feet

ATTACHED TO THOSE CHIC FRENCH CERTAIN AGE LEGS are their chic French certain age feet. Like their legs, chic French women's certain age feet are the result of good foot care and often professional help with regular pedicures. For the chicest of chic French certain age feet, the Paris "foot guru" is Bastien Gonzalez. His pedicures have also earned him the title of *artiste de la pédicure* and the reputation of someone who can make you feel as if you are "walking on clouds." Even wearing those mile-high French stiletto heels.

Though his heritage is Spanish, Bastien Gonzalez is French and a podiatrist medically trained for diagnosis and treatment of disorders of the foot, ankle and lower leg. His emphasis on a medically-based pedicure for prevention of foot problems explains how he earned his reputation. Beth Arnold who enjoyed one of Bastien Gonzalez's remarkable "true pedicures" reported on it for *The Huffington Post*.

His treatment [isn't] just cosmetic, as most are, but a medical curing of the feet, nails, and skin, plus a therapeutic foot and leg massage. His clients' feet would not just be attractive but also natural and healthy. Gonzalez took a preventive medical stance, which was to understand the origins of his clients' foot problems and to teach them how to better care for them.

Only his select clientele enjoy Bastien Gonzalez's pedicures, but he makes his pricey foot care products available for sale on his website. He also gives his advice on caring for your feet for free. Dry feet and toes well after bathing to prevent fungal growth. Use a foot balm and massage the feet nightly, particularly the fatty cushion at the bottom of the foot to give it back volume and suppleness. Massage the legs to help circulation and to minimize foot pain. Wear shoes that will adapt to your feet. If you wear very high heels, each evening do calf stretches and pull toes forward to relieve pressure on the joints.

One of the most frequently asked questions I received in the early days of the *Chic & Slim* website was how French women could wear high-heeled shoes with no hosiery. The answer, of course, is talcum powder. Almost everyone knows that now. It's another of Bastien Gonzalez's recommendations. The powder absorbs moisture and reduces shoe friction. Medicated foot powders offer even more benefits.

While chic French women do not often use colored polish on their fingernails, they do like it on their toenails. A clear red has long been the popular color. It was that red that made the original red sole on Christian Louboutin's stiletto heels, pricey footwear often found on chic French feet.

Just because a chic French women reaches certain age does not mean that she will begin wearing "comfortable" shoes as so many American women do. Though she may opt for a mid-heel such as those we saw candidate Segolène Royal wearing during her French presidential campaign. But with regular foot care and perhaps a little professional help, a chic woman of certain age has no need to give up her sexy high heels for orthopedic shoes.

Body

FRENCH WOMEN CHOOSE A VARIETY OF *SOINS*, care treatments for their head-to-toe beauty. But when they want to put the whole body back in shape or to relieve stress, they go to a spa, usually to one where they can experience *la thalasso*. Thalassotherapy (from the Greek word *thalasso* meaning sea) is the use of sea treatments for both preventing and recovering from physical and mental stresses. These treatments use not only the sea water, but marine mud, seaweed and algae as well as the bracing sea air and beautiful scenery of the seacoast to revive and beautify the body and elevate the spirit. There may be no fountain of youth, but the French think a week soaking in their French seawater, being slathered with their marine mud and wrapped in their seaweed at one of their *thalasso* centers is a good substitute.

Numerous internationally-known *thalasso* spas are found along the French coasts, particularly the Atlantic coast. They are also found along the Channel and the Mediterranean coast. Further inland, *balnéotherapy*, bathing in the waters from thermal springs, is regaining popularity as some of the long-established spas integrate anti-aging programs and programs for well-being after age 50 into their services.

During her adult years, today's chic French women of certain age likely will have chosen thalassotherapy for everything from stress relief to putting themselves back in shape after giving birth or gaining a few kilos. Customarily a French woman visits a *thalasso* spa sometime between the fourth and seventh month of pregnancy for future mommy care. She will have massages, relaxation sessions in pools of warm seawater and wraps with mud and algae so her body can absorb their important minerals. Her breasts will be given special treatments to keep them unaltered by pregnancy. She will receive facial treatments and advice on healthy eating during pregnancy. Then, when her newborn is around six weeks old, mother and baby return to a spa for more *thalasso*. In the *jeune maman* or *poste-natale*, young mommy or after-delivery program, the emphasis is on treatments to tone her body back in shape after giving birth. Mother and baby will have massages, and spend time soaking up the healthy nutrients from the warmed sea water. While mother is receiving her personal treatments, the spa will provide care for the infant.

At other times, to recover from an illness, or shape up her silhouette, or have special treatments for *jambes lourdes*, the chic French woman will have had other week-long or weekend treatments at a *thalasso* spa.

The menu of many *thalasso* spas show special programs for Slimming, Facial Beauty, Back, Anti-Cellulite, Light Legs, Balance and Nutrition, Back in Shape, Relaxation and Harmony, to name a sampling. But relatively few at the time of this writing list a special program anti-age. The explanation is that by their very nature most of the various thalassotherapies are anti-age. Especially those that treat facial wrinkles and bring relaxation and energy to the body or improve circulation. And since most spas do an initial medical evaluation of each client on arrival, any issues related to aging would be worked into their personal program.

One *thalasso* spa that does offer a special anti-age program is *La Thalasso de Roscoff* in Brittany. The spa's *bain de jouvence*, bath of youth, designed for both men and women age 40 and older is a six-day program that aims at remineralalizing the body, shaping and strengthening the body, and hydrating the skin. Beginning with a consultation with a doctor, the client would have one body scrub, 3 massages done under a water spray, 3 green tea body wraps, 1 firming massage with grapeseed oil, 1 lifting massage with argan oil, 1 reflexology of body and face, 3 jet showers, 3 hydromassaging baths, 2 sessions of calisthenics followed by a vitamin cocktail, 1 lifting facial massage, 2 sessions of Dermo V4 for the face, 1 gymnastic workshop for the face, the later which I interpret as likely being taught facial exercises to counter the effects of aging.

And if all that massage and wraps along with spraying and soaking in sea water doesn't set back the clock a little, what would?

Another spa that offers a specific anti-aging cure is *Thermes Marins de Monte Carlo*, one of the Riviera's most exclusive (and expensive) spas. When Anoushka Healy checked out the spa for the *Times Online* (UK) she noted the spa's old-style Riviera glamour and commented:

> It is a great place to people-watch as Italians in their towelling dressing gowns and sunglasses chatter into their mobile telephones, wandering among the elegant French women d'un certain age and the younger women from Russia who preen and pamper themselves in preparation for a night at the Casino.

When the interviewer for French *Elle* asked Italian actress Laura Morante, one of those auxiliary chic French women I have included in the book, what special pleasure she allowed herself from time to time, she answered a session of *la thalasso* at Quiberon.

Quiberon is one of the well-known *thalasso* spas in Brittany. If a session there is even half as restorative as their downloadable 36-page color brochure makes it appear, then one well understands the actress's choice. Of course as devoted to afternoon tea as I, the photo that I found most appealing was that of a young woman, her sessions with *thalasso* over for the day, seated on the terrace overlooking the sea with her book and afternoon tea.

Many recognize La Roche-Posay as the name of the French skin care company recommended by many dermatologists around the world. *Laboratories La Roche-Posay* are there in the charming spa town in the Poitou-Charentes region. All the company's skin care products contain the thermal water rich in selenium, silica and calcium known for its benefits for skin problems.

The *Centre de Balnéothérapie Thermale de La Roche-Posay* defines itself as a centre of Thermal Dermatology. For decades, people from many countries have come to this charming corner of France to take the spa treatments with its "velvet water." Many *balnéo* treatments are similar to those at a *thalasso* center, but using the thermal water instead of sea water. Like *thalasso*, *balnéo* is designed to help the client become more beautiful, care for the skin, lose weight, or simply relax and de-stress. All of the *soins*, treatments can be enjoyed à la carte, but programs are available organized around the same goals as *thalasso*: facial care, slimming, body care, *jeune maman*. And now anti-age.

A recently-established Anti-Age Unit offers a variety of programs that incorporate the spa's various massages, wraps, water treatments, skin analyses and medical consultations with the availability of a clinic that gives Botox, hyaluronic injections, peels, laser treatments, and Mesolift, a treatment that uses injections of anti-oxidants, vitamins and minerals under the skin to lift sagging skin and decrease wrinkles.

When I watched the informational video, once past the scenes of the beautiful location, the featured patient looked more like a New Yorker of certain age, than a French woman. A second patient that appears at the end of the video definitely looks like a grandmother from Iowa. When coffee is served to the patient at the end of her treatment, it's in a paper cup (very un-French) with a familiar-looking logo on the side. My thought was: this woman could be having this treatment anywhere in the USA. Perhaps this is purposeful and the Unit is catering to women who want to take advantage of a French vacation not only for *balnéotherapies*, but a little Botox and peeling too. Puzzling that the Anti-Age Unit lists the San Francisco based SkinCeuticals as their cosmetic partner. Why not La Roche-Posay whose laboratories are right there in La Roche-Posay? Or even another French skin care company?

VICHY IS A NAME EVEN MORE KNOWN around the world than La Roche-Posay. The city in the Auvergne is also the location of a thermal spa whose waters have been known since Roman times to bring health and beauty. The spa there has also added an anti-aging program for its clients.

Vita, designed for French-speaking Canadian women over 40, is a sister publication to Canada's *More* magazine. Not long after celebrating her 50th birthday in Paris, writer Louise Richer went to Vichy to check out its new anti-aging treatments at *l'Institut des Laboratoires Vichy au Spa thermal Les Célestins*. A preliminary skin analysis told her that her 50-year-old face had a skin age of 41. After this delightful news, Louise Richer continued with what she describes as 105 minutes of bliss. First a head massage, then a bath in the thermal waters, then, an exfoliation followed by a masque designed to boost cell regeneration. Her report confirmed my opinion that the four-hand massage done while warm water sprays down on the body is heavenly.

Vichy also offers a 6-day Anti-aging Beauty program as well as a similar Active 50s program designed for both men and women. I found it interesting to compare the two programs. No doubt because the anti-aging beauty program is designed for younger women, this program begins with a beauty status report. But the 50s program designed for those of certain age, begins with a medical consultation. Both programs provide skin diagnoses and dietary consultations. After these initial consultations, both get the "300 million new cells treatment." The name suggests something Frankensteinian, perhaps some sort of injection of cells from some exotic creature. A little further reading suggested to me something more benign: an extensive exfoliation, as I understood it, one that would cause one's own body to produce new healthy skin cells.

While the anti-age beauty received Cryotherapy and Thermo-sudation wraps, the active 50s have Vichy mud and Auvergne mud wraps. Mud wraps are obvious, but I have no idea what Cryotherapy or Thermo-sudation wraps are. Something beautifying apparently.

Those in both programs receive the two-hand shower massage and the Vichy hydromassage bath, but the anti-aging program has a Lipodraining jet massage and 50s has Lipodraining jet shower. I had jet massage years ago. Basically it's having your body pummeled with a jet of water from a high pressure water hose something the size and force of those used by firemen in fighting building fires. The aim is toning the body, particularly hips and thighs. Jet massage is apparently considered too force-ful for people in their 50s.

A client of the 50s program will have two IYASHIDOME sessions meant to mimic being buried in warm sand Japanese-style, but the anti-age beauty will get Celestins beauty treatments. As someone who has spent a lot of time on sandy beaches, I think the

IYASHIDOME would surely be pleasant while one was buried in the warm sand. But I can remember that no matter how carefully you showered when you came in from the beach, you would always miss some grains of sand hiding somewhere on your body. Gritty stuff, sand.

Both programs have Aqua-biking, very popular now in France. The exercise bicycle pedaled is underwater in a pool. Said to be excellent to tone thighs and to get rid of saddle bags.

Both Vichy programs include a Vichy spa drinking cure. Some additional treatments are included for both programs to make a total of 22 Vichy Thermal Spa treatments for the Anti-Aging Beauty and 19 for the Active 50s.

ONCE WE HAD MANY THERMAL SPAS in the USA where people went to take treatments based on the waters. Most have now vanished, though places such as Berkeley Springs, West Virginia, and Saratoga Springs, New York, are still in operation. The French have continued the use of sea water and thermal springs through the centuries for health and beauty, adding new treatments as science and technology progresses. Chic French women of certain age avail themselves of water therapies for rejuvenating their spirits and their chic French bodies.

Anne, your books are like mental chocolate truffles.
Merci beaucoup!
Judy

Menopause

IMPOSSIBLE TO WRITE ABOUT WOMEN OF CERTAIN AGE and not write about menopause. How do chic French women cope with the physical and emotional issues arising from this mid-life change in their bodies?

When hormone replacement therapy (HRT) became available several decades ago, French women and their doctors responded enthusiastically. The therapy known in France as *THS* or *Traitement Hormonal Substitutif* was widely prescribed. Then, in 2002, when the results of two major studies, one in the USA and the other in the UK, pointed to breast cancer and other risks associated with the use of the therapy, French doctors no longer so readily prescribed *THS*. Some French women elected to discontinue use. A number of those who had never taken the therapy decided when the need arose to find other means of relief from problems associated with *la ménopause*.

Today only an estimated one in three French women takes *THS* to relieve menopause symptoms. That is still substantially higher than the 20 percent of menopausal women the National Institute of Health figures estimate are taking HRT in the USA. Though it should be noted that the medications prescribed in French *THS* are not identical to those generally prescribed in the USA.

As for the American women who continue to take HRT, studies indicate a direct correlation between educational level and taking of HRT. The higher the education level of an American woman, the more likely she will take HRT. This should not surprise anyone. The higher the education level, the more likely the woman would be involved in work for which the physical symptoms of menopause would make it more difficult to do her work at peak performance. Any health risk would be offset by the necessities of her job.

SO IF ONLY ONE IN THREE FRENCH WOMEN of menopausal age today take hormone therapy, what do the other 67 percent do?

First of all, they take the guidance of their physicians. Following that guidance, or on their own, they may make use of water therapies. That Vichy Active 50s program that I wrote about in the previous section is designed to provide techniques and solutions for the less desirable physiological and psychological effects of menopause and andropause. (Apparently in France, men also are considered to go through a mid-life change that requires attention and treatment.)

In any case, the water therapies, both *balnéo* and *thalasso* are well designed to provide relaxation to deal with the emotional distresses of menopause. Other therapies in their programs work to mitigate the bodily changes such as increased problems with circulation and vein problems. All the nutritional and exercise coaching sessions incorporated into the programs offer help with diet and exercise, keys to alleviating menopausal symptoms.

The French have long found homeopathic remedies, essential oils and various nutritional and herbal remedies useful for all sorts of ailments. Likely many being used today for problems of menopause were those that were in use before the advent of the prescription *THS*.

The magazine *Femme Actuelle* provides its readers with extensive information on the *les médecines douces,* soft medicines, for *les bouleversements dans le corps des femmes,* upsets in women's bodies of menopause.

One exotic remedy for *les bouffées de chaleur,* hot flashes was *Lachesis Mutus,* a homeopathic tincture prepared in part from the venom of the Central American snake by that name. Those who are not enthusiastic about snake venom for their *bouffées* might try a massage with essential oils. The magazine suggests 2 drops essential oil of clary sage and 1 drop essential oil of peppermint mixed into two soup spoons (tablespoons in American measure) of a vegetable oil. Massage delicately into the lower back. Those wanting to add nutritional punch to their hot flash prevention, the magazine suggests increasing the amount of Omega 3 in the diet and limiting alcohol and caffeine.

The magazine also suggests additional homeopathic, essential oils, and nutritional aids for dealing with other menopause-related problems: emotional fluctuations, decrease in libido, weight gain, and bladder leakage. Though it might be noted that a recent study published in the *American Journal of Obstetrics & Gynecology* suggested that overweight and obese women by reducing their body weight a modest five to 10 percent (for instance, an 8-pound loss for a 160-pound woman) found a significant reduction in incontinence symptoms. That's good news because incontinence is a real challenge to chic.

One herbal remedy you do not find among suggested treatments for menopause in France is black cohosh, a popular herbal treatment for menopause symptoms in the USA. Curious, I went looking for a reason for this exclusion. The best answer I found was on the French language Wikipedia page for Menopause. Here it said studies have shown black cohosh has serious undesirable adverse effects on liver function. Anyone who has spent any time around the French know that they take the optimum functioning of their livers very seriously.

YET, FOR MANY CERTAIN AGE WOMEN the struggles in menopause are those of the spirit as well as of the body. How do chic French women cope with those?

In Bethany Ladimer's book *Colette, Beauvoir, and Duras: Age and Women Writers*, she gives an example from a short story "Menopause" by the French writer Marianne Servouze-Karmel in which the author describes a fifty-year-old-French banker, Suzanne, who "very consciously suffers from physical and emotional symptoms of menopause."

For her, the crisis most directly concerns her childlessness, for now she will never have a child, and her other family members are dead. After she observes from her window the nervous breakdown of another fifty-year-old woman, the resulting night of insomnia ends with her determination to be the child she never had and to offer maternal care to herself. She will find a lover and seek ways to relate to young people that will satisfy her emotional and physical needs.

While menopause may bring physical and emotional challenges, French women choose from a variety of treatments and solutions that make this time happy and productive. And, of course, chic and slim.

Food

WHEN I WAS LOOKING at the various *médecines douces*, soft medicines, recommended in that *Femme Actuelle* section for dealing with the problems of menopause, I was amused that when it came to nutritional advice for preventing weight gain in mid-life, the section just said to the readers, "You already know how to do this."

French women know the techniques for losing weight and staying slim. These techniques are basically the same for certain age as for other eras of women's lives. I have already discussed these techniques extensively in the other *Chic & Slim* books and on the *Chic & Slim* website *annebarone.com*. I will not repeat this information in this book. What I shall cover in this section on Food are additional aspects relating to food particular to certain age.

The first thing you need to know is that you cannot commit excesses in food and beverage in certain age that you did when you were younger. At least if you do not want to pay a high price in the way you look and the way you feel. Moderation might have been advisable when you were young. In certain age, moderation is a necessity.

You will see chic French women of certain age replacing morning or after dinner coffee with a *tisane*, herbal tea—

sometimes replacing both. Dinner wine might be diluted with mineral water. Or the wine replaced entirely with water.

Health problems increase in certain age. But many of these problems can be prevented, made less severe, or cleared up entirely by food and lifestyle choices. It's that simple.

The French are more likely than Americans to take this good food choices avenue toward good health, possibly because their national health care covers many preventative treatments designed to educate and encourage them in healthy food habits. Many health issues are related to excess consumption, and in France, excess is frowned on. In America, excess is considered a constitutional right.

My redneck brother, the one whose motto is: "If it ain't fried, I don't like it," has an increasing number of health problems requiring more and more expensive medications and treatments. But make any changes in his eating habits to relieve the problems? No way.

One very un-chic health problem of certain age is bloating related to intestinal gas. American drug store shelves are loaded with an astounding number of products designed to deal with digestive problems. Medical science relating to the digestive system assures us that most of these problems could be eliminated by moderate portions eaten slowly and chewed carefully and not washed down with such large amounts of liquids that the digestive juices are diluted beyond effectiveness.

Sometimes in certain age a food can be eaten with no problems as long as it is not eaten at the same time as another food. A simple solution here is a small notebook that serves as a food diary. If you find intestinal distress after eating a food, make a note of all the foods that you ate at this time. After keeping notes for several weeks, look for patterns. You might be able to eat a food without problems if you don't eat it at the same time as another food. If a food combination you love is causing problems, you may want to eat this only when you are alone. Of course for severe or persistent digestive problems, you should consult your doctor to make sure the problem is not something more serious than simple indigestion.

Hormone replacement therapy not only relieves *les bouleversements dans le corps des femmes* but even more importantly is taken to prevent osteoporosis. Unfortunately medications developed to deal with osteoporosis seem to have unwanted side effects, so there is a definite incentive for women who do not take HRT to follow a diet that helps prevent crumbling bones. A diet suggested by French dietician Florence Piquet to *Femme Actuelle* strikes me as being basically what we have come to know as the "Mediterranean Diet." Florence Piquet argues that dairy products are not the most useful sources of calcium and that a sufficient amount of this important mineral can come from calcium-rich vegetables, from nuts and from legumes such as chickpeas, lentils, beans, and from soy products. Though recognizing that it would be almost as impossible for a French woman to eliminate cheese entirely from the diet as to give up bread, the dietician suggests a limit of one small serving of cheese a day.

By the way, not only is the Mediterranean diet good in the prevention of osteoporosis, but research at Columbia University has found those who eat that Mediterranean-style diet have a 40 percent lower risk for developing Alzheimer's disease. Other studies have also noted reduced risk for memory loss when eating the Mediterranean way.

Medical science disagrees about whether metabolism, that process that burns food for body fuel, actually slows down when a woman reaches certain age and thus requires that she decrease the amount of food she eats to maintain healthy weight. Since metabolism is not something inflexible, but can be increased or decreased by physical activity, by food eaten, and some tests indicate by the mind, I think that in many cases it is not the metabolism that slows down in certain age, it's the woman.

My own experience is that I can eat the same amount of food in my 60s as I ate in my earlier years and not gain weight, but I must eat quality food to have the same level of energy as even five or six years ago. For years, for breakfast I could eat a 3-inch section of baguette spread with butter and an all-fruit jam with a cup of coffee or tea with milk and have all the energy that I needed until lunch time. Not any more. Certainly not if my brain is going to function efficiently for a session of writing followed by a couple of hours of gardening or household renovation before lunch mid-day. I have to be especially careful that I am getting sufficient potassium. For me, potassium seems to be a key nutrient for energy. Since I have always tested borderline anemic no matter how much iron-rich food I eat, I also must make sure I include a lot of iron-rich foods. I must be equally careful for quality in the other meals of the day. I have even become more careful in the choices for the small amount of sandwich or pastry that accompanies my afternoon tea.

If I lived in France, buying quality foods would not be as great a problem as it is here in the USA. (See Michael Pollan's book *Omnivore's Dilemma* or Eric Schlosser's *Fast Food Nation: The Dark Side of the All-American Meal* if you need more background information on the dismal quality of most of the food sold in American supermarkets.) Many of the agribusiness practices that produce low-quality and often unsafe food in the USA are simply against the law in France.

Also helpful are organizations such as EcoCert I previously mentioned in the Makeup section. EcoCert is primarily concerned with food testing and manages to test about 70% of the organic food industry in France and about 30% worldwide. The EcoCert certification is to even more stringent standards than that of the government. Concerned consumers can look to certification of groups whose standards they know and respect for the safest and highest quality food.

As I said earlier in the book, I consider the US Department of Agriculture certifications largely worthless since that department inspects such a minuscule amount of food eaten in the USA. As far as the FDA is concerned, that agency is hamstrung by inadequate staff, testing facilities and authority to do much about unsafe food. A new law recently passed for safer food is targeted by the new Conservative-controlled House of Representatives to be dismantled. We live in sad times when our elected officials vow to place the profits of corporations over the health and safety of the nation's citizens, particularly its children. Eating healthy and safe in the USA will likely become even more difficult and time-consuming and, no doubt, expensive in the future.

Perhaps this difference in the quality and safety of the food available in the USA and France helps explain the contrast in chic American and French women's approaches to food. We have, for example, fashion designer Norma Kamali in the *Yahoo Shine* article about how fit she is at 65 described as: "Looking 45." She tells her interviewer the secret is eating raw food and how much better she feels since she has given up bread. Don't look for a chic French woman who has given up bread. The French are about as likely to give up bread as they are to give up sex. A chic French woman of certain age might moderate her bread intake and choose some of the whole grain varieties offered by the bakeries, particularly the *pain aux céréales* now so popular. But never give up bread entirely.

In a *New York Times* article profiling the chic and active 99-year-old Esther Tuttle, she explains that for most of her adult life she has followed a Dr. Atkin's-like diet of meats and fats and very low carbs. (She does have a tiny slice of 100% rye bread for lunch.) But she never, never eats dairy. France is the country that prides itself in its more than 400 varieties of cheese. French women might moderate their intake of dairy for a specific health reason, but never give up cheese entirely. Nor yogurt of which they are fond, especially for a quick, easy supper.

The chic French certain age approach to food is perhaps best summed up by chic and slim French actress Leslie Caron, at 79 still making films and directing her *auberge*. She told writer Susan Spano: "I eat a little bit of everything." And that "everything" includes the wonderful fare prepared by her chef at her *Auberge La Lucarne aux Chouettes* in Villeneuve-sur-Yonne, France.

In most places and at most times,
appreciation of savor in food has usually gone cheek by jowl
with appreciation of beauty in women.
The pleasures of the table have a natural affinity with the
pleasures of the bed.
Waverley Root in *The Food of France*

La beauté de votre peau est le miroir de votre santé.

The beauty of your skin is the mirror of your health.

Stress

STRESS IS AGING. We do not need medical studies (though there are plenty) to tell us this. We can look in the mirror.

Chic French women are known for their calm serenity. And chic French women of certain age are even calmer, more in control, more self-assured than younger French women. No doubt this ability to resist the ravages of stress contributes to their ability to age gracefully and beautifully.

You have already seen in previous sections, treatments and products chic French women use to combat stress and to give them beauty that contributes to their self-assurance. The strong social safety net France has woven provides French women with a security that eliminates many of the stress-producing worries with which many women in the USA must constantly struggle.

French national health insurance and health care that rates among the very tops in the world not only take care of women's physical and emotional health, but foots the bill (if their doctor prescribes) for many treatments that de-stress and beautify. French women have guaranteed maternity leave and assurance that their job will be there when they return. They have excellent pre-natal, delivery and post natal care. (Didn't those *thalasso* treatments for pregnancy and for mommy and new baby sound

lovely?) Families have payments to help pay for household help
and other expenses with small children. French doctors make
house calls for sick children. France has a public pre-school system
that is unique in the world. Birth control and abortion are readily
available for everyone and subsidized for those of low income.
Should they lose their job, there is unemployment assistance.
Almost every neighborhood has excellent *instituts de beauté* and
salons to beautify and de-stress. For busy women with no time to
cook, there is healthy prepared food in easy shopping distance.
Public safety is strong, and if the rowdies get out of hand, the
French take steps toward laws that take away their citizenship. Six
weeks of annual vacation is guaranteed and there are numerous
official holidays in which one can relax and rejuvenate. Generous
pensions make for an enjoyable retirement. Good facilities are
available to care for elderly parents. The country is a wonderful
melange of beautiful natural scenery, splendid architecture, good
transportation, delicious cuisine and fine wine. The older woman
is valued and respected. If all this were not enough to eliminate
stress and bring serenity to chic French women of certain age, the
French are the highest consumers in Europe of anti-depressants.

But for those of us who do not live in France, but in countries
where the weak social safety nets we have are being dismantled—
and where the growing income disparity predicts an unhappy
and difficult future for those not in the highest income brackets—
women of certain age must find ways of dealing with that stress
that otherwise would only accelerate the natural changes taking
place in our bodies and minds. What to do? You might find a new
book useful.

Thea Singer, the author of the recently published *Stress Less:
The New Science That Shows Women How to Rejuvenate the Body
and the Mind* told Liz Jones in an interview for the *Daily Mail* (UK):

The most chronically stressed are women at mid-life:

their children are teenagers or young adults, their parents are old and perhaps needing care. They find they are having to earn money and provide for and care for all these different generations at a time when their bodies are getting older, when they are approaching the menopause and worrying about retirement. It is middle-aged women who are the most stressed-out beings on the planet".

Thea Singer is a science writer and her book explains what science has learned about stress and what it does to the human body. Her interviewer Liz Jones, who went through a hellish three years of stress, did an excellent job for her review distilling from Thea Singer's 300-page book, a summary of the how-to for women to deal with stress and even outwit the biological clock to look even younger than their age. When I read Liz Jones' summary I saw that most were things I have been advising you to do beginning with the first *Chic & Slim* book.

First of all, you don't diet. Diets don't work. (And, Thea Singer assures us, they stress and age the body.) You need to eat real food with quality nutrients at regular meals in moderate proportions. Exercise reduces stress, but you have to have a program that you enjoy and which fits well enough with your lifestyle that you can follow it on a regular basis. Likewise, I have encouraged you to get adequate sleep. Sleep becomes even more important (and often more difficult) in certain age than when you are younger. French women find short naps great for de-stressing and as a beauty aid. Many of the spa treatments aim at making regular sleep easier.

While I have never specifically suggested that you meditate, I have recommended Bellaruth Naparstek's guided imagery programs that are a kind of guided meditation. I have used her *General Wellness* and *Weight Control* for years and find they are the perfect way to relax and revive when I am feeling worn out mid-day. Less than 30 minutes with a program either on CD or on my iPod and I have new energy and renewed spirit. Sometimes when I am emotionally frazzled or very tired, too tired to even insert the ear buds of the iPod in my ear, I simply lie down and do deep breathing with my mind focusing on the breaths which constitutes a kind of meditation.

By example, I have encouraged you to be optimistic. Many of you have written letters and sent emails commenting on my positive attitude and ability to face setbacks with humor. Our economic situation today in the USA is difficult, and we have people running for public office (some even elected) who only a few decades ago not only would never have been on the ballot, they would been kept by their families in a back room under strong medication. But those who have studied American history know that the country has in several periods been "on its way to Hell in a hand basket," but still somehow the forces of common sense have regained control and we survived for a better day.

When my mother went to a nursing home and I packed up her house, I saw many photos, read many letters and saw much memorabilia of that period of the 1930s we call the Great Depression. I grew up hearing stories about how terrible things were during that time. But when I looked at the photos and memorabilia and read the letters and packed the items purchased during those tough times, I understood that things were difficult during the Great Depression, but people still had meaningful lives and some moments of joy. And they helped one another. And they helped people who were in even more difficult circumstances than they—even though they had little to spare themselves.

If we keep our heads, we can weather these current difficult days. Still, it might be a good idea to pack up and move to France, precisely what many Americans have always done in the past when things get looney in the USA. On the other hand, Canada is closer, and if you really want to speak French, there is Quebec.

Exercise

IN THE USA, TOO OFTEN EXERCISE is something one *should* do, but often one does *not* do. America has made convenience and ease such priorities, and the automobile so central to life, that opportunities for healthy exercise as an integral part of one's daily activities has almost been eradicated. To get exercise, American women often have to make a special effort.

Not so for chic French women.

Walking is still the way a great many chic French women exercise, and often this exercise comes as part of daily routine. Walking to public transport to take to work, walking for shopping, walking to the neighborhood *institut de beauté* or hair salon. Writer Tatiana de Rosnay says her exercise is that she tries to do all her errands on foot. Actress Laura Morante says she walks for exercise every day. One thinks of the 20th century French writer Colette who, certain age and suffering from arthritis, walked daily. When asked what exercise she did in bad weather, she said she walked in bad weather.

Recently in *The New York Times* there was an article on equality for French women. The photo with the article showed a 30-something French woman dashing across a Paris street. She has an infant in a snugly carrier, a toddler by the hand, and two active young boys dashing ahead. She is running in stiletto heels to take the children to day care *on the subway* before she goes on to the hospital where she is a physician. The article tells us that she will spend the day seeing patients at the hospital (in those heels) then make the homeward dash (one assumes the way she came: partly on foot, partly on the subway). French husbands do not help much with household chores so she will fix dinner for the family and prepare the four little children for bed. Does anyone seriously think this woman needs a gym membership for exercise?

Pilates and yoga are popular with chic French women of certain age. And a number do enjoy sports. Christine Lagarde, 55, the French finance minister, is a former champion swimmer. She swims several times a week and also enjoys biking and scuba diving. When Guinness Book of Records named 98-year-old French sisters, Raymonde Saumade and Lucienne Grare as the oldest living twins, Raymonde's daughter, Claudie Saumade, told CBS how exercise had always been part of her mother's and aunt's lives. "They have always been exercising. They were born in Paris in front of the Japy gymnasium. They started when they were 10-years-old, and they have done it ever since." She added that her mother played basketball until she was at least 67. Both twins had taken advantage of living near the sea for swimming. Jeanne Calment, the French woman who held the title of the oldest living woman at age 122 at the time I wrote the original *Chic & Slim*, rode her bicycle until she was 100. Not for exercise, but for transportation.

As you read previous sections, you saw how chic French women keep themselves in shape with those cold baths and self-massages for toning and aiding circulation. *Instituts de beauté* and spa treatments correct for figure flaws and give many of the same health benefits as exercise. But they do it without sweat and strain of jogging or workouts on machines. Machines are often involved, but they are those such as the Cellu M6 with its suction and rollers applied while one relaxes on a table. Then there are all those products sold in pharmacies and natural product stores that are swallowed or rubbed on to improve the figure.

Several things strike me about all the methods of exercise chic French women of certain age employ. They have either the element of utility or the element of pleasure. Walking to a place one needs to go, or walking for the pleasure of seeing beautiful and interesting surroundings. Any exercise done where they will be observed by others, particularly male others, a French woman of certain age is careful to look chic while she exercises. Walking in high heels or other attractive footwear. Swimming is in a flattering swim suit. (Mid-50s Segolène Royal was photographed at the beach in her bikini during the presidential campaign.) Pilates in a body-hugging leotard. These are good. But dripping sweat with feet clad in running shoes? *Non, non, non!*

Exercise is an essential ingredient for keeping you physically and mentally youthful in certain age. Not just medical research, but observation of our family and friends shows us the difference exercise can make at this stage of life. If you want to be healthy and attractive and have a brain that functions well for you in certain age, you must incorporate some exercise into your life. Regularly.

Your reason for exercise is not to stay slim. Exercise will help you stay slim, but exercise is only one of many factors in a successful campaign for a svelte certain age body. More important reasons are that exercise is essential for good physical health, to keep your brain working well, to reduce stress, to beef up your immune system to fight off disease, to aid sleep, to help cope with *les bouleversements* of menopause, to give you a more attractive appearance, and to put you in condition to enjoy life's joys and pleasures. Those pleasures certainly include good food and romance.

In her chapter on Stress and Exercise in her book *Stress Less*, author Thea Singer quotes authorities on exercise and aging. John J. Ratey, M.D. author of *Spark: The Revolutionary New Science of Exercise and the Brain* says: "Exercise is one of the few ways to counter the process of aging." And S. Jay Olshansky, professor at the University of Illinois at Chicago and first author of *The Quest for Immortality: Science at the Frontiers of Aging* who says: "Exercise is the only equivalent of a fountain of youth that exists today." Dr. Olshansky points out that the benefits of exercise are instantaneous. When you exercise, you feel better immediately.

While writing this book, when the work was flowing well there was always the temptation to skip my exercise session for the day. Just stay at the computer and keep writing. Most of the time I resisted this temptation—and benefited from coming back to the computer with re-energized brain and body. But the day I first attempted to write this concluding part of the Exercise section, I gave in and did only a few minutes of stretching late afternoon. I paid a price. My brain stalled. The writing became mush and at the end of the day I had to delete all I had written. In the evening my legs ached from too-long immobility. I woke in the night with an aching back from all that sitting at the computer with no exercise relief. Exercise is worth the time it takes.

How much exercise is necessary for certain age?

Just about all the medical authorities, including the official agency for such guidelines in the USA, the Centers for Disease Control (CDC), say we need at least 30 minutes of moderate aerobic activity such as a brisk walk at least six days a week to which you tack on at the beginning and end of your session a five-minute warm up and a five-minute cool down. Thirty minutes of vigorous aerobic activity such as running or jogging would suffice done three times a week. For really good health benefits, you would need to engage in double the amounts listed above. And, of course, before you start any new exercise program, you need to check with your health care professional to make sure you have no medical reason not to follow that particular program.

About the time I reached certain age, I read some exercise authority who said that for brisk walking, you needed 20 minutes to get your heart beat up and then an additional 20 minutes exercise to keep it pumping at that rate. When you tack a cool down on to this, it makes a 45-minute exercise session. That 45-minute session has usually been my minimum walk. But I often go beyond that when I am enjoying my exercise. Or when my blood pressure for one reason or another is elevated. Exercise, I have discovered is the absolute key to keeping my blood pressure normal in my mid-60s. Something I want very much because I do not want to take blood pressure medicine.

For many busy certain age women finding even a 30-minute segment five days a week can be difficult. Shorter segments squeezed into your day can bring benefits too. A friend who worked full time and had heavy family responsibilities could manage only 10 minutes on a treadmill before work, 10 minutes during her lunch hour, and 10 minutes in the evening. The three 10-minute sessions a day along with moderate, sensible eating helped her lose 40 pounds and dramatically reshape her body.

Like so many chic French women, the aerobic exercise in which I most often engage is walking. For me, at least when the weather is not impossibly bad, walking is pure pleasure. My daily voyages of discovery in my little queendom, or when I travel, as the best way to explore a new place.

But there are all sorts of fun alternatives for those for whom walking is not possible or who just don't like to walk, even on a treadmill while watching TV or listening to a good audio book. Putting that CD in the player and dancing, working out with an aerobics DVD, joining an aerobics class are three possible alternatives. Just find the exercise that is pleasure. And take a tip from chic French women, that no matter what exercise you do, you will enjoy it more and likely reap more benefits if you make an effort for chic in your exercise clothes. Baggy sweats may be comfortable. But they are not chic.

READERS COMMENT

I have been a regular visitor to your website since the year 2000, and I really enjoy your attitude, insight, and smarts on living the chic life with fun and gusto. You have been a role model for me of sorts.

Best wishes and thank you!
Stephanie

I was just telling a friend of mine about the Chic & Slim lifestyle. I told her that your books have done more for me than most of the spiritual self-help books I have read. Fully embracing the Chic & Slim lifestyle allows one to live happily in the now instead of constantly searching for happiness.

Merci,
Meredith

I just want you to know how much I enjoy your web site. You have given me great recipes, juicy gossip and encouragement to streamline and simplify my wardrobe and body. Your links to great articles have stretched out my self-imposed boundaries and enriched my life.

Jan *in California*

Sleep

NAPS ARE WONDERFUL for a beautifying and rejuvenating boost. Chic French women use them well for this purpose. But for healthy mind and body and avoiding the ravages of lack of sleep on your face, you need good sleep in longer stretches. You need about eight hours sleep every 24 hours.

Unfortunately, for certain age women, everything from hormonal fluctuations to financial worries to elderly parents needing care can prevent getting needed sleep. Healthy habits I learned from chic French women are useful in laying the basic foundation against sleep problems. Moderation in caffeine intake and eating (so no digestive problems), keeping alcohol limited, regular walks outdoors in the fresh air, regular hour of bedtime, sleeping with some fresh air in the bedroom, a relaxing settling into bedtime with some (not too exciting) reading. Staying slim is an asset too. Excess weight can cause sleep problems.

When problems with menopause or stress make falling asleep difficult, French women often find drinking a *tisane* (herbal tea) thirty minutes or so before bedtime useful. Chamomile and valerian are two popular ones. I enjoy chamomile, but not the taste of valerian, for me the more effective of the two. I prefer valerian in capsules available at a natural foods store. Valerian has been used since ancient times for insomnia. Not toxic and having few adverse effects, it is generally safe for occasional use.

When I was doing much international travel across time zones, the doctor's recommendation for a safe sleep aid to compensate the body clock was Benedryl, a brand name for the antihistamine diphenhydramin. But diphenhydramin makes me feel groggy the next morning. So I prefer valerian that leaves me clear-headed. The only time I choose the diphenhydramin is if I have been badly bitten (again) by fire ants or mosquitoes and the itching is interfering with sleep.

From a *New York Times* article on sleep, I learned it is a good idea to end computer use at least an hour before bedtime. The bright light from the screen can signal wakeup to your body making it more difficult to fall asleep. I had gotten into the habit of checking email and reading news right before bed. It was then taking me an hour or so of reading to feel sleepy. Shutting down the computer earlier, I find that my eyes are beginning to close before I have read more than a couple of paragraphs.

An excellent tip for solving sleep problems came from a reader comment to one of the *New York Times* sleep articles. Sometimes it is a pet that is interrupting your sleep. Cats are nocturnal and mine gets into phases where she prowls the house during the night. Last summer when she was waking me about three times a night jumping on and off the window ledge and doing very noisy cleanings about 3 AM, I fixed her own bed in another room and shut her out of mine. I slept through the night. At least until my neighbors next door began their morning door slamming.

If noisy neighbors are preventing your sleep, the first step should be to talk with them and ask they be quieter. This almost never solves the problem, but when you then file charges against them with the police, the officer will ask you if you tried asking the neighbor to be quieter. If you can say yes, the police are likely to be more sympathetic and helpful. But if the neighbors appear to be mentally disturbed or drug users, the police will understand why you did not talk with them.

When it comes to caring for elderly parents, when they are not sick enough to be hospitalized, they are sometimes well enough to make not-really-necessary demands out of childishness and fear about their condition. Sometimes for self-preservation you must be tough as in: "No, I will not wake up at 2 AM and 4 AM and walk you to the bathroom. You are going to wear this Depend. And I am going to get some sleep. Pretend you are an astronaut and your spacecraft is coming in for a delayed landing."

When you are so worried about finances or job loss, or other serious problems that you can't sleep, good lifestyle practices and a cup of herbal tea probably will not be enough to ease you into sleep. By the time I was 50, I had survived enough difficulties that whenever a new one arose, I felt confident that I had survived the others and I could survive new ones as well. This confidence keeps sleepless nights from worry at a minimum. I get the sleep I need to be able to solve my problems.

There was a time when, if something was nagging my mind so that I could not sleep, I would get put of bed and try to work though the problem. But even though I was awake, I was tired and unable to do my best thinking. Now, on a sticky note, I write down three actions I will take first thing in the morning to deal with the issue and post it where I will see it. This reassures my mind that something will be done, and I can generally fall asleep.

Chic French women of certain age understand the importance of sleep and make efforts to have both naps and sufficient night time sleep. You should do the same.

Work

ALL THE CHIC FRENCH WOMEN DISCUSSED in this book are still working. None, as far as I can learn, have retired. Though actress Catherine Deneuve, 67, who has over her career made more than 100 films, 16 since age 60, has said that she now may make fewer films than in the past. She would like to have some time to enjoy her garden (one of her passions) and her five grandchildren.

Even the oldest of the chic French women of certain age in this book are still working. Françoise Gilot, 89, is still traveling, still promoting the sale of her art works through media interviews and attending gallery shows of her paintings. Liliane Bettencourt has been busy the past year meeting with her financial advisors and lawyers fighting her daughter's efforts to have her declared incompetent over her gifts to a much younger man. At the same time she has weathered a scandal involving political donations to politicians in the highest levels of government. Interviews she gave to the media about the situation show a sharp older woman, far from incompetent, who knew exactly what she was doing and believed she had the independence to do it. As I write this, in the past week, the media has reported that Liliane Bettencourt has brought a halt to the incompetence declaration efforts and reconciled with the daughter, as well as come to a satisfactory outcome in the relationship with the younger man. The political scandal seems to have died down, and the effort now is to think in terms of the future of L'Oréal of which she owns 31 percent. A busy year of work for 87.

The French interior designer Andrée Putman, 85, continues a busy design schedule. Her Wikipedia page updated a few weeks ago recounts:

> Mme. Putman recently unveiled the Blue Spa at Bayerischer Hof hotel in Munich, the Guerlain flagship store on the Champs-Elysées and stores for Anne Fontaine in Tokyo, Paris and New York as well as private residences in Dublin, Miami, Paris, Rome, Shanghai, Tel Aviv and Tangiers. Most recently, she designed a 31-floor apartment skyscraper in Hong Kong, conveniently named The Putman.

Some chic French women once they reach certain age branch off into a new career direction. Actress Jeanne Moreau, now 83 and still appearing in films, turned to directing in her early 60s. Recently actress Fanny Ardant, 62, made her debut effort as film director. Her *Cendres & Sang* (Ashes & Blood) was praised by France's *Liberation* as "stunning, magnificent, beautiful and dazzling."

The most dramatic certain age career change of a chic French woman was that of my friend Mimi. Born in Paris, she was educated in Catholic boarding schools and the Sorbonne. As a young woman she married an American doctor and came to live in the USA. In certain age, the marriage failed. Her career as doctor's wife ended and her children grown, she set out to establish a new career. Since she was living in Texas, it seemed logical to this Parisienne to go into ranching. She bought land and cattle and moved into the ranch house. The venture was not a success. But she never regretted the experience. Later she was heard to say, "When I had my ranch . . ." and "On my ranch. . ." phrases that always play well in Texas.

Carine Roitfeld, 56, for 10 years the editor of French *Vogue* told her interviewer for the *Guardian* (UK): "When I was younger and the children were small, I was not working so hard. I was very lucky, because I had a husband who had a great company and was earning very well, so I had the liberty to raise my kids and not work every day." But she explained when the opportunity came, she had the energy and appetite for it. "I think if I had had to work too hard when I was younger, I would not love it so much now. It's like when you squeeze a lemon too hard, you run out of juice. Me, I have plenty of juice." Certain age may be the time for some women to launch their most successful career. It might be the best time. As I was finishing this book, Carine Roitfeld announced that she would soon be leaving *Vogue*. In her mid-50s, she is looking forward to yet another new career.

Barbara Strauch, author of *The Talents of a Middle-Aged Brain* assures us that the middle-aged brain is better than a younger brain at inductive reasoning and problem solving. It also gets the gist of an argument better and is better at sizing up a situation and reaching a creative solution. Barbara Strauch assured Tara Parker-Pope in an interview in *The New York Times* WELL blog that our brains in middle age are better than in our 20s because they have had time to build up all sorts of connections and pathways. And as for keeping the brain at its peak performance, the best thing we know for that is good physical exercise.

Jacqueline Kennedy Onassis, an American woman very French in her approach to style and life, began a new career in certain age. At 46 she began a career as a literary editor and continued in that work until only a few weeks before her death at age 64. Two recent books deal with Jackie's career as editor. In reviewing those books Celia McGee wrote:

The two books both make the point that Mrs. Onassis's lifelong passion for reading, and her two decades in publishing, reveal much about her as a person: the intellect behind the fashion plate, the analytical mind behind the famous face. The little girl whom Mr. Kuhn describes sneaking books out of her mother's library, and, at Miss Porter's School, not letting her roommate, Nancy Tuckerman, interrupt her reading, grew up to spend more years as an editor than as first lady and the wife of a Greek shipping tycoon combined.

When the former first lady lost her battle with cancer and her son John Kennedy, Jr. came out on the steps of her home to announce to the media and the world keeping vigil that his mother has passed away, he gave assurances that she had died peacefully surrounded by her family, her friends and her books. Books were Jacqueline Onassis' passion and her work. For certain age women today, work is often as important as friends and family.

In Joseph Conrad's *Heart of Darkness*, his character Marlow is struggling with the near impossible task of putting a decrepit old steamboat in working order so he can get take it up an African river. Marlow has this to say about work:

I don't like work—no [one] does—but I like what is in the work, the chance to find yourself. Your own reality—for yourself, not for others—what no other [human being] can ever know.

Women have always worked. Today many of us actually receive money and recognition for the work we do. But more than money and acknowledgement, for many of us, the greatest rewards of working are those discoveries we make about our own abilities and our own worth.

Boundaries

WITHHOLDING INFORMATION ABOUT ONESELF for mystique should not be confused withholding information as a means for setting boundaries. Mystique is about allure. Boundaries are for necessary protection.

When the unmarried French Justice Minister Rachida Dati became pregnant, she refused to name the father. An article in a December 2008 *US News & World Report* stated:

> Ironically, the news that unmarried Dati, 43, is expecting a baby in January has been the least of the issues in a country in which about half of all babies are born to unwed mothers (with some couples opting for civil partnerships rather than marriage). But the rounds of speculation over the father, whom she chooses not to identify, has brought an element of farce with awkward denials of paternity from various men, including a former Spanish prime minister and a prominent sports figure.

If a bunch of nervous men wanted to issue denials of paternity, that was their business. But for Rachida Dati the identity of her daughter's father was personal information the public was not invited to share.

The little girl is now a toddler. Rachida Dati has been replaced as Justice Minister and dispatched to Strasbourg as a Member of the European Parliament. As far as I know, papa's name is still a secret.

French actress Isabelle Huppert has always been cautious about revealing personal information. In an interview with Robert Chalmers for the *Independent* (UK) she declined to answer the question of whether her parents were still living even though this and much additional family history was public information. The interviewer easily learned the answer from other sources, but assumed that the actress had chosen not to answer because to do so might have invited questions about her early childhood she did not wish to discuss.

We all have areas of our personal life it is stressful to discuss. And unless, as Martha Stewart learned the hard way, we are responding to investigators whom the law requires we give exact personal information, we have no obligation to reveal that information.

Actress Kristin Scott Thomas told a *Daily Mail* interviewer that she found interest in her love life "boring and scummy." She said she would not talk about the subject, because it sets you up for people to prod and pry and speculate.

Not only for well-known actresses, but for other women as well. If you give people unlimited information about yourself, it does set you up for people to prod and pry and speculate. If you don't give them bait in some areas of your life, then they can't fish for information it might complicate your life if they knew.

Chic French women of certain age are especially adept at setting boundaries to the information they share with others. Learning to be skillful at managing your own information can save you much stress and unhappiness. In certain age as in any age.

Mystique

MYSTIQUE, AN AURA OF MYSTERY, has long been a potent weapon in chic French women's arsenal of allure. By the time she reaches certain age, a chic French woman is extremely skillful at using mystique to her advantage. Especially in their fine art of developing a romantic relationship.

Today a mystique is harder to create and maintain. We live in an age when every cellphone has a camera. An age of instant communication. Google. Wikipedia. Facebook. Twitter. The 24-hour news cycle. People who go on national television and not only tell the most intimate details about themselves, but about everybody else they know. Ex-lovers write tell-all books. Paparazzi stalk the streets. Yet the basic fact remains: when people know "too much," when there is no mystery left, when there is nothing more to learn, people lose interest. Chic French women of certain age today still believe mystique has value and try to maintain some 21st century version of one.

How does this work? At the most basic, a woman does not talk constantly about herself. She does not reveal every fact about herself. She leaves something to be discovered, yet at the same time she must demonstrate that there is something there worth engaging with long enough to discover. If a woman of certain age is attractive, it helps focus attention sufficiently that others might put out the effort of discovery.

Several decades ago I read a description of French mystique at work. It has remained in my mind as a classic demonstration of this chic French women's technique at work. My memory credits the French artist and writer Françoise Gilot, but since I did not at the time note the source of the information, I cannot be absolutely positive.

In any case, Françoise Gilot on a visit to the USA in 1969 was invited to a dinner party at which Dr. Jonas Salk was also to be a guest. She told her interviewer Suzy Kalter in a 1979 *People* interview that she had been introduced to Dr. Salk first at a business lunch. But the example of mystique that I remember came at a dinner party a few days later there in La Jolla, California.

In those days, Dr. Salk was a medical superhero. His vaccine had conquered polio, the dreaded disease that had killed and crippled so many Americans including a US president.

Françoise Gilot was as well-known as Dr. Salk. First as a successful artist, as well as the woman who had lived for nine years with Picasso and who was the bestselling author of *Life With Picasso* published five years previously. Friend of Matisse whose work had influenced her own art. Additionally she was a beautiful woman just approaching certain age.

Picasso, Matisse, her life on the French Riviera, her life in Paris, art, all the topics this woman could have interjected into the conversation at the dinner table. But in the description of that party I remember, throughout the dinner, Françoise Gilot purposely listened to others, but made no conversational contributions herself. Several days later, Dr. Salk phoned inviting her to tour the Salk Institute where Françoise Gilot told *People* it was "love at third sight."

Would this man have phoned and offered the private tour of the Salk Institute if there was nothing more to learn about this woman? Françoise Gilot did tell *People* about their conversation during the tour, "I thought Jonas and I were from two different worlds but when we started to talk we knew we had so much in common."

Françoise Gilot and Jonas Salk were married in 1970 and remained so until his death in 1995.

Ben Brantley writing in "Whatever Happened to Mystery?" in *The New York Times* reminds us:

When we first fall in love with people, they always seem remote, unattainable. Holding on to love after you've crossed the divide between you and the object of your desire is a chapter in achieving maturity; it's what marriage is supposed to be. But there's a part of us that needs to keep falling in love with the girl in the mists in the distance or the boy riding away on a horse.

A savvy chic French woman of certain age manages to be the real woman right there, but to always keep a part of herself elusive, "the girl in the mists."

L'Amour

The thing about France—the way women are perceived—is not that once you're past 40, you're past IT. On the contrary, experience is very attractive. We like seeing a woman with lines, we like seeing a woman who looks like she has experience; that's exciting. A pity there isn't a little more of that elsewhere.

The above statement made by Actress Kristin Scott Thomas in an interview with Kristin McCracken published in *The Huffington Post* points to a salient fact about French women of certain age: the appreciation of their experience and intelligence, not to mention their well-maintained beauty makes them desirable not only to men their age and older, but to younger men as well. No surprise when France's regional health observatory states that 85 percent of French women in their 50s, and 63 percent in their 60s are sexually active. Ample evidence suggests many French women continue their amorous activities past 70.

Why do French women stay amorously active, often with younger lovers, past the ages at which many women in other countries no longer have the interest or the opportunities for lovemaking? No one has come up with the definitive answer.

Observing and studying what other say about French women through the years, I offer several theories as to why l'amour remains a part of French women's lives.

Theory: *Tradition.* The French can look back in history to many famous French women no longer young who had love affairs. For one, Diane de Poitiers, the favorite mistress of French Renaissance King Henri II. Diane was 18 years older, and their affair began when Diane was almost 40 and continued until the king's death at the time she was 59. In her book *Seductress,* Elizabeth Prioleau tells us that Minette Helvétius, the 18th century certain age siren who so charmed our American representative Benjamin Franklin, after the death of her husband: "created herself anew. She gave her homes to her daughters, bought a cozy estate in the Paris suburbs, and threw herself into senior seduction with gusto."

In the 19th century, Aurore Dupin who wrote under the pseudonym George Sand, in certain age had numerous lovers. The older she became, the younger George Sand's lovers.

Theory: *Pleasure.* The French put great importance on pleasure and *l'amour* is very pleasurable.

Theory: *35-Hour Work Week and Early Retirement Age.* This gives the French much leisure for *l'amour* that workaholic Americans don't have. I am not sure if the person who suggested this idea to me was serious, or simply expressing anti-French cynicism.

Theory: *Wine and Good Food.* A pleasant meal is relaxing, and with a moderate amount of wine, likely to put one in the mood.

Theory: *French Women of Certain Age Stay Slim.* Not only is a slim, well-toned body sexually attractive (especially when alluringly attired), but excess weight and certainly obesity can lead to health problems that can result in diminished libido or simply not feeling well enough to be active. My theory, however, gets a refutation hit from the 20th century French writer Colette.

When Colette was 47 she scandalously seduced her 16-year-old-stepson. Their affair lasted five years. Colette had been a beautiful young woman, but by her late 40s she was fat, and her hennaed hair was a frizzy fright. Looking in this stage of her life according to Elizabeth Prioleau like "Hagar the Horrible with a bad perm."

Judith Thurman researching *Colette: Secrets of the Flesh* asked René Aujol who had known Colette and the stepson at the time of the affair how could the fat, almost 50-year-old woman have been attractive to the young man. His answer was: "Colette was desirable, oh, extremely. One could easily imagine sleeping with her. She had a powerfully seductive aura that's not obvious from her photographs." Judith Thurman comments: "Fat women, when they are fit, are often much sexier half-naked than dressed, and Colette was still limber and superbly muscled with Venusian breasts and the biceps of a discus thrower."

Theory: *Avoiding Women-only Activities.* I have observed that American women—and these are totally heterosexual women—tend to become involved in women-only organizations. Religious retreats, camping trips, women's organization conferences, women's business groups, exercise groups, book discussion groups. The list seems endless. French women have little interest in any activity at which there were no men present. This enables French women to keep their social skills fine-tuned so when they do meet someone of interest, they will be able to move the relationship forward.

Theory: *Action Against Weight Gain and Loss of Libido.* Reading French women's magazines, I sense two chief concerns for French certain age women today are weight gain and loss of libido. They take action against both. There's that lingerie that makes them feel good about themselves. And all those massages and beauty treatments and sessions at spas that not only make them more attractive, but de-stress as well. And when what is available in their pharmacies, at their *instituts de beauté* and their spas isn't enough, they get help from their doctors. French women don't just bemoan their problems. They take action to solve them.

Theory: *No Guilt*. Lisa Armstrong's piece on French women in the *Times* (UK), made an interesting point about guilt.

This is another myth—that French women are all busy having affairs. Statistically, they're no more likely to have affairs than we are, but they probably are less anguished about their extramarital hobbies. In the national psyche an affair is not necessarily a cause for angst, soul-searching and divorce, but a pleasing diversion that can save a marriage. *Ménage à trois* is French for happy compromise. Given that sex is always going to beat *crème de la mer* and the gym as youthefiers, and that feeling cherished is (almost) as good as Botox, is it any wonder age fails to wither them.

Theory: *More Tolerance*. French women's greater tolerance for their husband's and their partner's extra-relationship affairs works to their advantage. How exactly? In an interview with Diane Johnson about her novel *Le Divorce* on *Penguin.com*, the author commented on the different attitudes toward infidelity in France and the USA.

There seems to be a fundamentally more realistic attitude in France that this common form of transgression occurs— in about the same proportion in both societies—but [Americans] are more hypocritical and more upset. No one likes to be a cheated-on spouse, but where the American wife gets a divorce, a French wife gets a trip to the Seychelles or pearls.

The affair which was likely not serious is forgotten and the marriage is preserved. Instead of becoming a lonely divorcée, the French woman retains her in-house lover.

Theory: *French Attitude Toward Women's Sexual Appetite*. In Judith Thurman's Colette biography she makes this observation:

> At least since the Puritan revolution, and probably since the reign of the first Elizabeth, ambitious Anglo-Saxon daughters have been taught that their greatest worldly leverage—the route to influence in art, politics, or anywhere in the public sphere resides in abstention. Despite misogynistic laws and traditions, French culture ultimately prizes and respects sexual appetite and daring in women and, as these women age, values their prowess and wisdom—one reason Colette would become a national treasure.

Judith Thurman wrote the above in the early 1990s. In the past two decades attitudes in the USA have undergone dramatic change. While there have been aggressive abstinence programs aimed at preventing pregnancy and sexually transmitted disease in teenagers, I do not think anyone today is seriously suggesting to ambitious adult American women who wish to reach the highest levels of success in the arts, politics or business that it would be to their advantage to appear to have no interest in sex. Quite the opposite. The times, they have changed.

A woman is never more beautiful than in a black skirt and pullover on the arm of the man she loves.
Yves Saint-Laurent in an interview with *Elle*

Style

The French didn't believe that true chic could be attained much before the age of 40. They were convinced it took a long time to learn the art of dressing and to develop an individual style . . . by then, when a woman's looks were beginning to fade she had to have chic or she had nothing.

Those words by journalist Alice-Leone Moats, quoted in Penelope Rowlands' wonderful fashion history *A Dash of Daring*, recalled a time before the Second World War. Today, with all those skin care products, spa and medical treatments, hair color, and other rejuvenation means we discussed in previous sections, things are not quite that desperate for French woman of certain age. It is not "chic or nothing." But chic is a still an invaluable asset for women no longer young — of any nationality.

In the previous *Chic & Slim* books I detailed the elements of chic French personal style. That effective combination of neutral colors, good design, natural fibers, simple lines, quality materials, perfect fit, and small workable wardrobes all worn with minimum accessories serves chic French women all their adult lives, evolving and perfecting as the years pass. In this book we look specifically at chic French certain age style and at some chic French women who showcase it.

Style in France today is becoming more casual. Given the times, this seems inevitable. But casual can be chic. Think Audrey. No one showed us casual chic better than the 20th century style icon actress Audrey Hepburn.

Two chic French women who do casual chic well (and no doubt who inspire others) are model and designer Inès de la Fressange, 53, and French first lady Carla Bruni Sarkozy, 43. They and Audrey Hepburn share body type: tall and thin. Here is a disadvantage of casual: more formal styles do a better job hiding figure flaws and other imperfections.

Inès de la Fressange, was a top model in the 1980s, a time of more formal dressing that she told Lisa Armstrong of the *Times Online* (UK) was an uptight and heavy time of "red lipstick and pearl earrings the size of cupcakes." But, she says, fashion was easier then. "There was more to hide behind. Now you have to have perfect skin and amazing hair, because it can't be too [styled]. And [white] teeth."

Earlier, in the 1960s, when women were still wearing hats and little white gloves, hats hid any certain age thinning hair and gloves hid age spots on hands. A well-designed dress could hide too-ample thighs and a bit too much tummy. Less-to-hide-behind today, however, is offset by the freedom to mix genres: an army-surplus coat with ballet flats. And to mix expensive with budget: designer belt worn with a khaki work shirt. Still you have to accept that in certain age you can't wear some things that you wore in your 20s. Flabby arms should avoid sleeveless, and skin tones often demand that neon pink should be declined in favor of a more flattering rose shade.

The article in the *Times Online* (UK) is a profile of Inès de la Fressange written in June 2008 when she was about to be awarded the French *Légion d'Honour*. The blogosphere was abuzz with suggestions that strutting down a runway and designing clothes (even if she had been Marianne, the face of France, from 1989 until 2000) might not be what Napoleon Bonaparte had in mind when he established France's highest honor. But argued Lisa Armstrong:

> So Inès, with her outstanding services to looking thoroughly damn stylish in an utterly inimitable French way is a more than deserving candidate. Plus, she's 50. This detail is important because de la Fressange is wearing her age in a way that seems possible only in France, which is to say, she's not trying to look as though she's 30.

In that last sentence is the essence of chic French certain age style: Dressing to look chic, not dressing to look young. Aiming for an ageless, timeless beauty.

At the same time Inès de la Fressange, whom many fashion observers in many countries now feel epitomizes French chic and elegance, assures us that while no longer wearing outfits she wore when younger, she would never go to a shop for 50-year-old women. What surprised me about this statement was I did not realize they had shops for "older women's clothes" in France. Who buys these? Tourists and non-French residents? I can't remember ever seeing French women wearing the type of older women's clothes you see in the USA. Certainly none of the chic French women of certain age we are discussing in this book.

Because I ordered a housecoat for my mother after she went to the nursing home from an American company that specializes in clothes for older women, I now regularly receive not only their catalogs, but those of several other similar companies. Glancing through the pages, I can never imagine chic French women of certain age wearing those synthetic, shapeless outfits: skirts with elasticized waists, overblouses, and loose mid-thigh jackets designed to hide tummy bulge. Chic French women don't need to hide tummy bulge when they are slim and their bodies well-toned.

If chic French certain age women do not wear elastic-waist skirts with boxy jackets, I do notice in cool weather French women in their 70s and 80s make marvelous use of walking length coats with beautiful scarves in the neck worn with tailored pants or slim knee length skirts and low-heeled, knee boots.

Men have no problem with casual chic. When Mark Anstead interviewed Kristin Scott Thomas for a *Daily Mail* article about her latest film, he noted with approval that she was "wearing a plain white blouse and jeans. Her style is the relaxed chic of her French adopted homeland."

Paloma Picasso and her French physician husband have two homes, one on Lake Geneva in Lausanne, Switzerland, and the other in the Palmeraie area of Marrakech, Morocco. Dana Thomas visited Paloma Picasso at her Marrakech home for a profile for *Harpers Bazaar*. The writer described the Tiffany jewelry designer's casual wardrobe:

Her Moroccan wardrobe is chic but distinctly comfortable: flowing colorful caftans in the summer and, on cool winter afternoons, soft, ample sweaters and slim trousers made for her by a local tailor. She keeps her jewelry, such as her ropes of lapis lazuli beads and long chains of hammered gold beads from her Tiffany collection, in a shallow green ceramic Moroccan bowl.

In her role as wife of France's president, Carla Bruni Sarkozy has earned approval both for casual and more formal fashion choices. Making an official visit either alone or with her husband to an outdoor site, you are likely to see her casually chic in slim black pants and a dark long-sleeved boat-necked top and flats with no accessories, not even earrings. But she is equally successful on formal occasions. Hilary Alexander, Fashion Director at the *Telegraph*, was one of many voices of approval of the ensemble Mme Sarkozy wore on the state visit to Britain in March 2008.

In dressing for her arrival at Heathrow, Carla Bruni-Sarkozy, demonstrated a political savvy which belied her brief tenure on the country's fashion throne. From "tête to toes", her ensemble bore the marque of Christian Dior, one of the most revered names in French fashion. But it was designed by an Englishman, John Galliano, couturier-in-residence at the famous maison on Paris's Avenue Montaigne. The outfit comprised a high-waisted coat in Dior grey – the colour most associated with the fashion house. It was accessorised with a matching beret, slightly tilted to one side to show Mme Sarkozy's signature demi-fringe. The coat was cinched with a wide, black leather belt, which emphasized her slim figure. Mme Sarkozy deliberately chose flat, black leather ballet pumps to detract from the height differential between her statuesque 5ft 9in and her husband's 5ft 5in, and carried — in black, leather-gloved hands — the latest entrant from the Dior 'accessory stable', a shiny black leather handbag, called The Babe.

This is perhaps the point to mention gray. Another change that I have observed in French fashion is that gray is the new chic French black. I was forcefully struck by this reality observing the audience at French *Elle* magazine's *Etats Généraux de la Femme* conference. In that audience made up of France's outstanding women in politics, journalism, arts, science and education, every woman it appeared was dressed in gray, even those of West African and North African origins.

My impression was confirmed recently by none other than French designer Jean Paul Gaultier who told the *Telegraph*:

"People think that everyone wears black in France; in fact they all wear grey."

For chic women of certain age, gray is good fashion news. Black, though chic and slimming, is a stark color. Black can make many certain age faces look "like an Italian widow," as the phrase goes. That is the reason, when wearing black, chic French women of certain age wear those scarves or wide choker necklaces. They put a more flattering color between the black and the certain age skin tone.

Gray can range from a dark charcoal to that blue-hued "Dior grey" of Mme Sarkozy's coat. Gray in tweed incarnation is classic and classy. Gray is a very Paris color.

There was a time when it seemed that chic French women of certain age would wear their suits and dresses—and certainly their high heels—even for casual events. Today they seem to have mastered casual chic without losing their chic Parisienne edge.

In Leslie Caron's 2009 autobiography *Thank Heaven,* she writes about donning jeans when she was doing chores during the renovation of the old buildings that became her charming *auberge.* But when Susan Spano interviewed Leslie Caron for *The Los Angeles Times,* Leslie Caron arrived far more formally dressed. "She had driven down from the French capital, where she lives, and arrived at the *auberge* looking like the quintessential Parisienne, dressed in a chic brown jacket with a gold lapel pin, with her little white lap dog in tow."

This is perhaps the point to mention brown and "what looks best on you." Note that it doesn't matter that "everyone" in France is wearing gray. Leslie Caron wore brown. Chic French women have the confidence, some say arrogance, to ignore fashion and wear what they please if it meets the criterion of making them look attractive. As someone with eye and skin coloring for which brown is a better choice than either black or gray, and whom navy blue makes look as if I have jaundice, I champion this French confidence.

Black is often mentioned as the signature color of Carine Roitfeld, for 10 years the editor of French *Vogue*. Though it should be noted that she does wear gray—and other colors. But she is definitely another chic French woman who, even as top editor at the most Parisian of French fashion publications, has the confidence to make her own fashion choices based on her fashion philosophy and personal style rather than on the trends she may be showcasing in her magazine. Not just in the matter of the color *du jour*. When designer handbags were bringing in revenue for *Vogue*, Carine Roitfeld still determinedly refused to carry one. (Where does she carry her lipstick? you ask. She does not wear lipstick.)

When discussing her personal style with Amy Larocca of *New York Magazine*, Carine Roitfeld defined the parameters of her casual chic: "Me, I wear a lot of Japanese piece [s] mixed with a bit of classic Hermès and Prada. Even though jeans suit me, I never wear jeans." Though it might be noted there is a Google Image of Carine Roitfeld wearing a slim blue jeans denim pencil skirt. She added, "I love the combination of a masculine piece with a feminine piece. It's very French, it's very sexy. It's my culture. It's the way I was raised."

Later in a conversation with Eric Wilson for *The New York Times* runway blog Carine Roitfeld explained the design of French *Vogue* and revealed personality traits of the chic French woman. She said that in French *Vogue* there was a "sense of beauty," a "sense of luxury," and what she called a "sense of craziness." That "craziness," however, reportedly went over the line into vulgarity and repulsiveness in the December 2010 issue and was a factor in Carine Roitfeld's departure from the editorship of French *Vogue*.

According to a report by Cathy Horyn who covers the French fashion scene for *The New York Times*, French *Vogue*'s advertisers were not amused by a photograph of "a pair of elders groping each other in a smear of lipstick and neck wrinkles." Nor by what Franca Sozzani, the very chic certain age editor of Italian *Vogue*, described as little girls "wearing heavy make up, sexy clothes, posing in poses that are outrageous for their age." Though she did not name the publication specifically, Franca Sozzani's comments are generally considered a criticism of the French *Vogue* December issue that included such photos. As the chic Italian editor concluded in her blog: "If what's beautiful depends on your opinion, what's ugly just repulses you."

However provocative the images that appear in French fashion publications, certain age French chic generally stays within the boundaries of good taste. As readers of fashion publications, certain age French women are generally more tolerant of provocative images than in the USA. But when it comes to dressing their own bodies, any provocative elements will be done with a subtlety that will delight, not repulse.

RACHIDA DATI, 45, THE FIRST WOMAN OF ARAB DESCENT to be given a key ministerial position in the French cabinet, has her own version of casual chic. She arrived for an interview with Elizabeth Day for the *Guardian*'s Observer wearing black leather pants, stiletto boots, gold hoop earrings and bright red lipstick. Elizabeth Day was particularly struck by the black leather pants and perhaps found them a more surprising fashion choice for Mme Dati than they were. The journalist likely was not aware that black leather pants have long been a wardrobe staple for chic French women, not only for young women, but for chic women of certain age. (After all, the certain age women are the ones most likely to be able to afford those pricey pants.)

The no-nonsense, but supremely chic, Michèle Alliot-Marie, 64, who replaced Rachida Dati as Justice Minister in Sarkozy's cabinet was photographed (in a full page photo, no less) for *Paris Match* in March 2005 wearing black leather pants at the time she was France's Minister of Defense. In any case, Elizabeth Day did see the principal significance of the high-priced designer fashions this daughter of poor, illiterate North African immigrants believes she has earned by education and hard work and which have generated much criticism for her.

Her clothes, it seems, go to the very core of Dati's identity; they provide both a means of self-expression and a symbol of her success – a sign of how far she has come from her impoverished start in life. She has said frequently in the past that being well turned out "is a question of showing respect towards others", an opinion that echoes Sarkozy's own conviction that there is nothing wrong with displaying the fruits of hard-won success.

Would Rachida Dati's critics be happier perhaps if she dressed more like another daughter of poor North African immigrants, feminist and government official Fadéla Amara, 46, whose chic appears to be more moderately-priced?

WORDS ARE LIMITED in what they can tell us about chic French certain age style. Images are needed. Fashion magazines have long played an important role in showing women chic style. But as Inès de la Fressange told Carola Long of the *Independent* (UK) today it is "impossible to find a woman who is more than 30 years old in magazines. It's like being older is hidden, there's no one for women to identify with."

But not so long ago, in fashion magazines, women of certain age saw plenty of fashions on women they could identify with. The celebrities featured on its pages were women of certain age.

Elsie de Wolfe, the American interior designer, was chosen in 1935 by Parisian couturiers as "Best Dressed Woman in the World" for her "high standard of taste" and "timeless elegance" as biographer Jane S. Smith explained. Elsie was 69 at the time. She may have been older. Elsie fibbed about her age a lot.

The quote at the beginning of this style section about French women over 40 needing chic taken from Penelope Rowlands' *A Dash of Daring* was from a section of the book discussing *Vogue* in the 1930s, both the French and American editions.

The magazine wasn't aimed at the youth market. Refreshingly, there wasn't such a thing, or at least not one that mattered. Fashion magazines targeted the older woman, giving tips for giving one's gray or white hair an elegant look, presenting a portfolio of styles with the sage headline "To Age Gracefully Is an Art." There were no tight faces, no desperately starved bodies in evidence.

Today you are seeing more older women in fashion magazines than only a few years ago. When in 2009 Jean Paul Gaultier brought the unlifted, un-Botoxed then 51-year-old Inès de la Fressange back to the runway to model his collection, it wasn't a stunt. M. Gaultier, certain age himself, was recognizing that there are many chic women of certain age with money interested in good design. It might be smart to show them how his designs could look on one in their age range. Karl Lagerfeld, another certain age designer, also saw the wisdom of this and settled his decades-old dispute with Inès de la Fressange and brought her to the runway for his own show.

Today anyone with a computer and a reasonably fast Internet connection can access an enormous amount of images of chic French certain age style. To begin, you can type the name of the French women of certain age discussed in this book into Google

Images. For most, you will find dozens of images that will give you clues to their chic. If, studying these images, you decide to make your own certain age style more chic French, I would suggest you consider the wisdom in the following:

In an interview published in March 2009 in *Interview Magazine*, Hamish Bowles, the European Editor-at-Large for *Vogue* stated:

I am absolutely crazy about Mainbocher's clothes. I think they are so subtle, the detailing is so extraordinary, and they are so unbelievably evocative of such a particular time and place and milieu and lifestyle, of absolute subtle luxury. Even his work from when he had his couture salon in Paris through the '30s—it has a kind of brisk edge to it and a crispness and a precision that is completely American. You can really see why a client like Wallis Windsor would have been drawn to his clothes, and why she became so emblematic of his work. It needs a client who really understands Europe but has a kind of brisk, no-nonsense American edge.

When I read the last line of this quote, I thought about what I was trying to communicate in this section on chic French certain age style. I believe you need to study and understand that French certain age style, but rather than trying to develop a personal style that is a copy, you should bring your own particular edge that reflects who you are: American, Canadian, Australian, British, Czech, Austrian, Singaporean, Chinese, whatever you are. Make your certain age chic uniquely yours.

Être Unique Avant Tout
Above All Be Unique

Aging Beautifully

IN CERTAIN AGE, DIANE DE POITIERS became the favorite mistress of the French Renaissance king Henri II. The monarch, though 18 years younger than Diane, remained devoted to her, and she remained his trusted advisor and companion, until his death a quarter century later. When Diane herself died six years after Henri at age 66, she was described by contemporaries as "having the figure and complexion of a woman of 30."

I opened *Chic & Slim Toujours* with the comment: *The further into your 60s you are, the harder it is to look 29. Not impossible. Just more difficult.*

In her mid-60s, Diane de Poitiers was said to look 30—not 29. Yet, considering that the 16th century lacked Botox, AHA peels, Retinol and all those other products and techniques helping women look youthful today—and that the Renaissance was an age when women, especially aristocratic women of certain age, were usually plump—then, being as wrinkle-free and svelte as a woman of 30 is indeed an impressive accomplishment.

Through the centuries many French women have demonstrated the ability to age gracefully and live full and vital lives long after the half century point. Diane de Poitiers is only one of many historical role models for chic French certain age women today.

You find many of Diane de Poitiers' beauty and style techniques still practiced by chic French women today. You find other parallels between Diane and today's chic French women as well.

Like many chic French women we have discussed in these pages, Diane was well-educated, not only in scholarly subjects, but in *savoir faire* as well. While Diane de Poitiers used her influence to promote the arts and intellectual endeavors of the French Renaissance, chic French women today not only support the arts and intellectual life of France, but many are the creators of today's art, literature, and films.

Like many chic French women today, Diane de Poitiers was not a great beauty. But she was so clever about her personal style and personal care that she convinced others that she was beautiful. Writings by her contemporaries and biographers tell us that Diane did not use the cosmetics of the time that ruined so many women's complexions. Like chic French women today, Diane concentrated on skin care. She created from natural products a sort of beauty masque against wrinkles. When outdoors, she employed that 16th century version of sunscreen: a black velvet mask that ladies wore that also protected against scratches from tree branches when on horseback. Diane was also said, when alone, to sleep propped up on pillows to prevent creasing her face.

Diane wore only black accented with white. These neutrals not only flattered her hair and skin, but gave her a unique personal style in a time when others in the court wore bright colors. Her clothes always fit her slim body perfectly. Perfect fit is another element found in the personal style of chic French women today.

Diane de Poitiers believed in the benefits of bathing and exercise. She was said to rise each morning, and even in the bitterest of winter, to bathe in cold water. Her belief in the importance of bathing is documented by the number of paintings done of Diane in her bath, some for which we are assured she posed. The most famous of these is the one done by French Renaissance painter François Clouet that now hangs in the National Gallery of Art in Washington, D.C.

In the Clouet painting we see Diane de Poitiers in her bath, her perky breasts on full display. But interestingly there is on the table beside her a bowl of fresh fruit. Though cold water toned the body and improved circulation (benefits that chic French women seek in cold baths and all that water therapy today) Diane also recognized the relationship between healthy food and beauty, as chic French women do today. Once she had bathed, Diane took her exercise spending two to three hours on horseback. Most chic French women today, however, will choose walking, biking, swimming or Pilates. They will also avail themselves of massages and other therapies that keep the body toned and shapely. Like Diane de Poitiers, chic French women see keeping body and mind beautiful and healthy as a lifelong process.

Her Royal Highness Princess Michael of Kent, a direct descendent of Diane de Poitiers, gives an excellent portrait of this French Renaissance woman and the French court during Diane's lifetime in her book *The Serpent and the Moon*. In the book's conclusion the author writes:

> Diane de Poitiers' legend lives on, not only because we see her today in the guise of her image as goddess created by the great masters of the French Renaissance, but because she was a woman of independent spirit who made an art of living the highest quality of life while preserving a youthfulness of spirit, body, and personality. She was an enchantress who inspired an unpromising youth to become a splendid king. That he loved her all his life, although she was twenty years his senior, is proof of her enduring mystique.

My aim in this book is to give you examples of chic French women from the past as well as the present so that you might, whatever your age, live the highest quality of life. That you would preserve a youthful spirit, body and personality that would not only give pleasure to those who know you, but serve as an inspiration as well. And that, with the example of chic French women, you would cultivate an enchanting mystique that would endure all your years.

Start now. Whatever your age.

Chic French women do not wait until problems become noticeable to begin their efforts. Healthy lifestyle habits are the foundation of a chic and happy certain age.

The earlier you begin, the more likely you will age beautifully like those chic French women.

The earlier you begin, the more likely that you will remain chic and slim *toujours*. Forever.

Vive les femmes d'un certain âge!

Resources

NUMEROUS WEBSITES AND BOOKS provided information useful to writing this book. Wikipedia and Google Search, along with Google Images and Google Books were especially helpful. Google Translate helped out when my rusty French was stumped. YouTube provided videos of several chic French women.

Many of the chic French women of certain age discussed in this book have a Wikipedia page or their own website. You can find links to these websites and Wikipedia pages with an Internet search using your search engine of choice. Many of the women have versions of their Wikipedia pages and personal websites not only in French, but other languages as well. Wikipedia's list of alternate languages is in the left hand navigation column. Other webpages may list the name of the language, or they may have the image of a country flag to identify the link. These are generally very small and often located in the upper right corner of the webpage.

The websites of French women's magazines were also valuable in providing information for this book. With their archives of articles and images, they can provide you with a wealth of additional material about topics discussed in *Chic & Slim Toujours*.

Even if you do not read French, you should be able to navigate the websites with easily recognizable link labels: *Mode, Beauté, Santé* (Health) *Shopping*. The images alone provide useful information about clothing and hairstyles. You will recognize many product names as those with which you are familiar.

Magazine websites I found useful were: *Madame Figaro, Femme Actuelle,* French *Elle,* French *Vogue,* French *Marie Claire, Paris Match* and *L'Express.* Italian *Vogue* (in English) has excellent articles as does *Vita,* a Canadian publication in French.

France24.com, Suite101.fr, Amazon.fr, Sephora.fr, rue89.com, fnac. com, college-de-france.fr, evene.fr, auFeminin.com and *linternaute.com* websites were also helpful.

The US magazines *Harpers Bazaar, People, Scientific American, D* (Dallas), *Harpers, Marie Claire, Business Week, US News and World Report,* and *New York* magazine provided information. *BooksinCanada.com* and *theTyee.ca* provided information about Nancy Huston.

The websites of colorist Christophe Robin and foot guru Bastien Gonzalez provided helpful care information. *YosemiteVeinCenter.com* provided explanations of hand vein surgery. *RestorationMed.com* provided explanations of popular esthetic treatments.

The French newspapers *Le Figaro, Le Parisien, France Soir, Libération* and *Le Monde* provided background information.

Several newspapers in the UK cover French topics well. I found useful information on websites of *Daily Mail, The Guardian, Times Online, Telegraph, Independent,* and *BBC News,*

In the USA, the best coverage of France and chic French women is *The New York Times,* particularly in articles by Elaine Sciolino reporting from Paris. Less frequently you can find articles about French women in *The Los Angeles Times. The Huffington Post* covers France and French culture at *www.huffingtonpost.com/news/france. The New Orleans Times-Picayune* profiled Françoise Gilot in article and video. *CSMonitor.com* profiled Marie NDiaye.

The websites of cosmetics companies provided information about the companies and their products. You can learn more about these companies and products on these websites, and in some cases, learn the location of a store in your area that sells their products. Mentioned in this book are Cattier, USA Weleda, Boiron USA, Dr Hauschka, Clarins, USA Mevita, USA L'Occitane en Provence, Leonor Greyl, Nuxe, Sisley, Lancôme, L'Oréal and Garnier. *Beautorium.com*, an online retailer for natural and organic products with USA distribution, has useful information about a number of products discussed in this book.

Websites of beauty institutes and clinics in France and the USA provided information about spa and medical treatments. You can learn more about beauty treatments in France on the websites of Dr. Daphne Thioly-Bensoussan, the *Institut des Jambes* in Rennes, the Spa Mosaic at the Hilton in Paris, the Anti-Age Unit at La Roche-Posay, the *Ville de La Roche-Posay*, the Active 50s program at Vichy, *Clinique Saint Aubin* in Toulouse. In the USA, you can learn about the clinic in Abilene, Texas, on the website of The Cosmetic Surgical Center of Texas.

The websites of The Sartorialist, WebMD, National Institutes of Health (NIH), Christine Valmy, and Renee Rouleau also provided information.

Books provided useful information about chic French women's beauty treatments and other topics discussed in *Chic & Slim Toujours*.

- Leslie Caron. *Thank Heaven*. Viking, 2009.
- Catherine Deneuve. *Up Close and Personal*. Orion, 2006.
  Linda Dannenberg. *The Paris Way of Beauty*. Simon & Schuster, 1979.
  Diane Johnson. *Le Divorce*. Dutton, 1997.
  Nancy Huston. "Dealing With What's Dealt" *The New Salmagundi Reader*, Spring/Summer 1995.
  Susan West Kurz. *Awakening Beauty the Dr. Hauschka Way*. Clarkson Potter, 2006.
  Bethany Ladimer. *Colette, Beauvoir, and Duras*. University Press of Florida, 1999.
  Princess Michael of Kent. *The Serpent and the Moon*. Touchstone, 2004.

Elizabeth (Betsy) Prioleau. *Seductress*. Viking. 2003.

Waverly Root. *The Food of France*. Knopf,1958.

Penelope Rowlands. *A Dash of Daring*. Atria, 2005.

Thea Singer. *Stress Less*. Hudson Street Press, 2010.

Jane S. Smith. *Elsie de Wolfe*. Atheneum, 1982.

Christine Valmy. *Christine Valmy's Skin Care and Makeup Book*. Crown, 1982.

For more information about these and other resources for *Chic & Slim Toujours*, visit the *Chic & Slim* supporting website *annebarone.com*.

Merci Beaucoup

From its beginning *Chic & Slim* has been a joy—and a struggle. Without support from numerous generous people, the struggle to explain French techniques for living chic and slim would have defeated me. For this particular *Toujours* effort, my greatest debt is to my son John. Without his support you would not have the *Chic & Slim* books nor website. From financial support to editing, to manual labor on *Chic & Slim* headquarters, his contributions, done without compensation, make the difference.

Nancy in Knoxville has made helpful financial contributions to the operating costs of the *Chic & Slim* website. If you enjoy the website, you owe Nancy your gratitude. My chic Canadian friend's plethora of delightful French-flavored gifts though the years has provided creative inspiration and much pleasure. Vicki in Friday Harbor's elegant Christmas messages each year have provided support and served as icons of the thoughtful communications that arrive from *Chic & Slim* readers.

Chic & Slim Toujours owes its existence to reader requests through the years for a *Chic & Slim* book specifically designed for women of certain age. Your insightful sharing of concerns for women to remain healthy and attractive in this stage of life suggested the topics discussed in this book. My thanks for your questions and comments.

Finally, I am truly grateful to those chic French women of certain age, past and present, who provide us such wonderful role models for living well and aging beautifully.

Merci beaucoup!
Anne Barone

YOUR TOUJOURS THOUGHTS

YOUR TOUJOURS PROJECTS

be chic

stay slim

toujours

Lightning Source UK Ltd.
Milton Keynes UK
175578UK00002B/68/P

9 781937 066093